TROUBLED CHILDREN

TREATMENT C   **6001074556**   \T: A Developmental Approach
by James F. Masterson

PSYCHOPATHOLOGY: Contributions from the Biological, Behavioral, and Social Sciences
edited by Muriel Hammer, Kurt Salzinger, and Samuel Sutton

ABNORMAL CHILDREN AND YOUTH: Therapy and Research
by Anthony Davids

PRINCIPLES OF PSYCHOTHERAPY WITH CHILDREN
by John M. Reisman

AVEF___ MATERNAL ___ A ___ of Schizophrenic
Devel___
by Al___ ___

│ Student

INDIVIDUAL DIFFERENCES IN CHILDREN
edited by Jack C. Westman

EGO FUNCTIONS IN SCHIZOPHRENICS, NEUROTICS, AND NORMALS: A Systematic Study of Conceptual, Diagnostic, and Therapeutic Aspects
by Leopold Bellak, Marvin Hurvich, and Helen A. Gediman

INNOVATIVE TREATMENT METHODS IN PSYCHOPATHOLOGY
edited by Karen S. Calhoun, Henry E. Adams, and Kevin M. Mitchell

THE CHANGING SCHOOL SCENE: CHALLENGE TO PSYCHOLOGY
by Leah Gold Fein

TROUBLED CHILDREN: THEIR FAMILIES, SCHOOLS, AND TREATMENTS
by Leonore R. Love and Jaques W. Kaswan

RESEARCH STRATEGIES IN PSYCHOTHERAPY
by Edward S. Bordin

TROUBLED CHILDREN:

THEIR FAMILIES, SCHOOLS AND TREATMENTS

LEONORE R. LOVE
University of California at Los Angeles

JAQUES W. KASWAN
Ohio State University

with

Daphne Blunt Bugental
University of California at Los Angeles

A WILEY-INTERSCIENCE PUBLICATION

JOHN WILEY & SONS, New York • London • Sydney • Toronto

WITHDRAWN

Copyright © 1974, by John Wiley & Sons, Inc.

All rights reserved. Published simultaneously in Canada.

No part of this book may be reproduced by any means, nor transmitted, nor translated into a machine language without the written permission of the publisher.

Library of Congress Cataloging in Publication Data:

Love, Leonore R. 1921—
 Troubled children.

 (Wiley series on personality processes)
 "A Wiley-Interscience publication."
 Bibliography: p.
 1. Problem children. 2. Child psychotherapy.
I. Kaswan, Jaques Waldeman, 1924- joint author.
II. Bugental, Daphne Blunt, joint author. III. Title.
[DNLM: 1. Child behavior disorders. 2. Child behavior disorders
—Therapy. WS350 L898t]

RJ499.L69 362.7'4 74-12232
ISBN 0-471-54788-3

Printed in the United States of America

10 9 8 7 6 5 4 3 2 1

To the families who participated in this study

And To Our Own

Series Preface

This series of books is addressed to behavioral scientists interested in the nature of human personality. Its scope should prove pertinent to personality theorists and researchers as well as to clinicians concerned with applying an understanding of personality processes to the amelioration of emotional difficulties in living. To this end, the series provides a scholarly integration of theoretical formulations, empirical data, and practical recommendations.

Six major aspects of studying and learning about human personality can be designated: personality theory, personality structure and dynamics, personality development, personality assessment, personality change, and personality adjustment. In exploring these aspects of personality, the books in the series discuss a number of distinct but related subject areas: the nature and implications of various theories of personality; personality characteristics that account for consistencies and variations in human behavior; the emergence of personality processes in children and adolescents; the use of interviewing and testing procedures to evaluate individual differences in personality; efforts to modify personality styles through psychotherapy, counseling, behavior therapy, and other methods of influence; and patterns of abnormal personality functioning that impair individual competence.

IRVING B. WEINER

Case Western Reserve University
Cleveland, Ohio

Preface

The 10 years of work reported in this book had two major goals. One was to identify characteristics of family and elementary school environments that seem related to children's personal and social effectiveness. A second goal was to develop and evaluate a consultation-type intervention designed to mobilize parents' and teachers' problem-solving skills in dealing with children's psychosocial difficulties. The developmental, clinical, and social aspects of these issues were examined through an integrated program of study that used both laboratory and field research methods.

Part I of this report examines the family and school environment of 120 children from 10 elementary schools located in widely varying socioeconomic areas. Within the family, we examined the patterns of verbal and nonverbal behavior. In schools we obtained data about the children's classroom and playground behavior. Actions and reactions of children could then be compared in both settings.

All data were analyzed in three ways. One compared the behavior and social context of children with serious adjustment problems with control children who showed no major difficulties. A second analysis was in terms of the socioeconomic backgrounds of the families. The third compared family and school data of referred children in relation to the specific type of problem manifested: aggression, hyperactivity, social withdrawal, or poor attention control.

Part II of the book describes the development, application, and evaluation of a "self-help" intervention made available to the adults in the troubled children's daily lives. The results of this experimental intervention, Information Feedback, were compared with outcomes of two standard treatments for children's behavior problems: psychotherapy for the child and counseling for the parents.

In this work we have drawn heavily on many disciplines. In turn, we believe that our results will be of use to colleagues and students in the many fields that deal with the growth, education, and treatment of children. Investigators interested in patterns of family behavior, parental role characteristics, parent-child relationships, and communication (nonverbal as well as verbal) within the family unit may have special interest in our methods and results, as may those concerned with the evaluation of novel as well as standard types of psychological intervention.

Inevitably, the results of a complex project cannot be presented without technical detail, but much of the statistical material in this report appears in appendices, and we have tried to present our findings in words as well as in numbers.

From the outset of this study, personnel in the Los Angeles school system gave unstintingly of their time. Dr. Berdine Jones of the Los Angeles County Schools offered early encouragement and support. Dr. Thomas Reece and Mrs. Louise Pierce (successive Superintendents of the Los Angeles Unified School District Elementary Area West during the project years) provided the backing necessary to make our work possible. Dr. Donald Kincaid (then Supervisor of Elementary Guidance and Counseling for the Los Angeles City Elementary Schools) and Maxine Ewers (then Coordinating Counselor for Elementary Area West) supplied guidance in the planning and implementation of this study; their counsel was literally a cornerstone of our work. The principals, counselors, and teachers in each of the 10 participating schools earned our gratitude for integrating many additional demands into their already burdened schedules. Their basic goodwill and concern for the children with whom they dealt were impressive.

The staffs of the UCLA Fernald School and University Elementary School permitted us to try out, repeatedly, the early forms of our instruments.

The participating therapists from the Los Angeles professional community, both psychologists and social workers, maintained admirable tolerance for research requirements while holding firmly to their clinical commitments. The graduate students in the UCLA Psychology Department Clinic, again both in psychology and social work, were equally flexible, reliable, and professional. Our thanks are due all these clinicians, too numerous to list.

Both of us have been integrally involved in all aspects of this study, from its inception through the completion of this report. We have enjoyed a genuine and equal partnership. But throughout this decade of collaboration, we have benefited inestimably from the contributions of many colleagues. It is a pleasure here to signify our indebtedness to these numerous contributors and to identify the most direct participants in our work.

Dr. Eliot Rodnick, as a co-director, provided invaluable consultation in planning the original NIMH demonstration and research applications and was an integral co-author in an early description of the project.

Dr. Lewis Ellenhorn helped in the development of the Adjective Rating Scale and in initiating analyses of videotapes during the first funded year of the project.

Dr. Daphne Bugental, joining the project in its second funded year, made numerous major contributions. She developed and reported a number of analyses of the videotaped family interactions. She was responsible for processing the change measures in the outcomes of treatments, and provided important technical consultation in many aspects of this work. We have reflected her significant role in the project through associate authorship credit in this report.

Dr. Armand Alkire played a major role in the development of the Family Communication Task, participated in providing Information Feedback consultation services, and also assisted in the early stages of data organization.

Evelyn Cohen, M.S.W., was responsible for all initial contacts with clients, and was instrumental in arranging the recruitment of parent counselors and the provision of supervision for social work students.

Dr. Alice Seeman helped develop initial measures of school behavior and coordinated the first year's data gathering at the schools.

Bette Overman took over these school liaison functions thereafter, as well as assuming full responsibility for all contacts with the control families and for much of the organization and processing of project data.

Judy Klusza, our computer programmer, was also responsible for much data processing.

Carol April, Ruth Cline, Diane Failla, Robert Giannetto, and Janet Wood headed a long list of research assistants; this list must include our dedicated project raters.

Drs. Harold Pepinsky, Daphne Bugental, and Armand Alkire and Ms. Bette Overman provided helpful comment on an early version of this report. Ruth Kaswan and John Love were our supporters, critics, and unofficial editors through the whole period.

This work was made possible by generous support from NIMH Demonstration Grant #1R11-MH-14770 and MH Small Grant #19695, UCLA Research Grant #2713, and UCLA Psychology Research Grant #1284. Our sincere thanks are expressed to all concerned. Computing assistance was obtained from the Health Sciences Computing Facility, UCLA, sponsored by NIH Grant FR-3.

Leonore R. Love
Jaques W. Kaswan

Los Angeles, California
Columbus, Ohio
July, 1974

Contents

CHAPTER 1

Introduction

The work described in this book had two major objectives. The first was to explore differences in the family and school environments of children who were seen as "disturbed," as compared to those considered "normal" by their elementary school teachers, counselors, and principals. The second goal was to develop and evaluate a psychological intervention for children's difficulties that focused on mobilizing the self-help capabilities of significant adults in the child's daily life, at home and at school. The effectiveness of this experimental intervention, termed Information Feedback, was compared with that of two widely used treatments for children's maladaptive behavior: Child Psychotherapy and Parent Counseling.

ORGANIZATION OF THE REPORT

This introduction contains an overview of the background, goals, and methodology of the project; Chapter 2 details some demographic, socioeconomic, and psychological characteristics of the study sample. This includes two groups of families: *(a)* 91 families of children 8 through 12 years old who were perceived by elementary school personnel as needing psychological treatment for serious social and emotional difficulties, and *(b)* 29 families whose children were described by teachers as functioning adequately. The "control" children were chosen to match a randomly selected third of the troubled children on the basis of age, sex, race, general intellectual capacity, socioeconomic level, and classroom teacher; in other words, they were chosen to be as similar as possible to the referred children except for their social and emotional behavior. All the children came from the West Elementary School District of Los Angeles. By means of careful selection of schools the children came from a wide range of socioeconomic backgrounds.

Chapters 3, 4, and 5 report measures of the children's interpersonal environment (family and school) in relation to the behavior of the two groups of children. Whenever possible, parallel sets of measures were used in fami-

1

ly and school settings. Within the family, two kinds of verbal reports of behavior were used (questionnaire responses and adjective ratings), and two samples of actual behavior were obtained (audiotapes of responses to a Family Communication Task and videotapes of family interactions in a standardized setting and sequence of events). School data consisted of teachers' verbal reports (questionnaire responses and adjective ratings), children's grades, and judgments (adjective ratings) made by trained observers viewing the children both in the classroom and on the playground. Analyses of results highlight comparisons and relationships between *(a)* the referred and control groups of children and their families; *(b)* the two interpersonal environments, family and school; *(c)* the types of behavioral difficulty manifested by the referred children (aggressive, hyperactive, socially withdrawn, or distractible behaviors); and *(d)* family socioeconomic levels. Chapter 6 integrates the results described in the preceding three chapters.

In Part II of the report, "Treatments," the effectiveness of three types of intervention for the referred children's behavior problems is evaluated. Two standard clinical treatments were investigated: psychotherapy for the child and professional counseling for the parents. Both of these treatments generally were based on psychodynamic formulations. The experimental intervention (Information Feedback) centered around the collection and feedback of data depicting the child's interpersonal experiences at home and in school. It was hypothesized that this information would serve to trigger parents' and teachers' change-producing efforts.

In the provision of these services, for the purpose of comparative evaluation of outcomes referred children and their families were assigned to the three treatments at random. Effectiveness of the clinical interventions was determined in terms of pre, post, and follow-up measures of the child's behavior at school, the situation in which his difficulties had been identified. Outcome criteria included systematic collection of school grades and teacher appraisals over a period of time, as well as repeated observation of the child at school by trained observers. Changes that were demonstrated in videotaped family interactions and verbal reports of family members were investigated as supplementary indices of altered behavior within the family.

Chapter 10 in Part II provides a description of the procedures and the hypothesized processes involved in the experimental Information Feedback intervention. The final chapter takes a critical look at some of our procedures and suggests directions for work in the future. Appendices A and B provide methodological and statistical details for the concepts and findings reported throughout.

BACKGROUND OF THE STUDY

The work reported here began almost 10 years ago. It grew out of concern about the limited range of conceptions and interventions available to help troubled children. Although societal, interpersonal, and individual influences were all recognized as contributing to children's difficulties, interventions current at that time consisted largely of psychodynamic treatment of the child and often one parent, usually the mother. The child's problems were seen as inhering largely in the way he processed his experiences; treatment therefore focused on those mechanisms. Mothers were seen concurrently to help them resolve their own intrapsychic difficulties and to increase their understanding of the child's problems. Fathers were often interviewed to enhance the therapist's knowledge of the child's background but were usually considered unavailable for continuing involvement, for either economic or psychological reasons.

School visits were sometimes made, and teachers consulted, but the primary emphasis again was on the child's psychological state, with his actions and interactions seen as consequent to his inner dynamics. Teacher's concerns were mobilized, but since the child's disturbed behaviors were defined as mental health problems requiring professional treatment, such contacts often made school personnel more tentative and hesitant in their interactions with difficult children than they had been before.

Professional focus on treating the child resulted in part from the fact that parents and teachers often did not seem to make (or maintain) the behavioral changes prescribed in therapeutic recommendations. Such failures were interpreted as reflecting inadequate flexibility or motivation for change on the part of the adults. Like many other clinicians, we gradually came to recognize that one intrinsic problem in this area was to a large extent ours, not our clients'. When we began to take into account the basic differences in social, cultural, and personal values in different client groups, and between some of our clients and ourselves, we recognized that our recommendations and judgments had often been unrealistic and overly simplistic. To the extent that they were based on the values of a specialized professional subculture (Pollak, 1956), they often failed to fit the psychology of the client. They therefore could not be expected to be useful to him, however valid and even self-evident they appeared to us. It seemed that means were needed to provide assistance for people's psychological and interpersonal difficulties that would involve minimum challenge to their personal and social standards, and minimal imposition of our value systems onto theirs.

As the size of the population seeking clinical service increased, the range of sociocultural backgrounds of clients broadened. For both reasons, the need for interventions other than "treatments" became evident. Procedures were needed that would focus on and maximize people's coping abilities, in contrast to identifying disabilities or pathologies for professional remediation.

In short, along with many clinicians in the decade of the sixties, we were concerned about the growing evidence pointing to the limited effectiveness of traditional clinical techniques, the scarcity of professional manpower, and the high cost of therapeutic services in proportion to growing social needs. In this context we reassessed our basic assumptions about psychological dysfunction in children and the implications of these concepts for effective intervention. We increasingly concentrated on the child's interactions with the adults in his daily life as critical in promoting or inhibiting his adaptive behavior, and we came to view these same adults as the appropriate focus for change efforts when children's behavior seemed disturbed.

The child's psychosocial effectiveness in general appeared to depend to a large extent on his experiences with the adults in his home and school environments. It seemed that a rote socialization process was ordinarily carried out by well-intentioned but inadequately informed parents and teachers. The defects in information which we identified were not those of educational or psychological sophistication, but rather represented a lack of specific information about the adult's own behavior and its consequences for the child.

As we studied families, it became evident that many parents paid little systematic attention to interpersonal phenomena on any except a subjective "feeling" basis. Interpersonal experiences between family members were usually not regarded as objective content to be paid attention to, noted, compared, or thought about. Behavior was not observed or processed in terms that would make it potentially subject to problem-solving approaches. In our context it seemed that interpersonal functioning might be improved if behavior could be recognized as related to the identifiable interactions that elicited it. Problem solving within familial interactions might be enhanced by making concrete, specific information about mutual perceptions and behaviors available to family members—and by facilitating the experience of taking an objective, rather than subjective, point of view while considering their interactions.

In our observations, adults usually seemed to have a generally benign intent toward children who depended on them, despite the many angry and insensitive behaviors they exhibited. Indeed, their negative, hostile, and ambivalent actions often seemed to represent their own frustration at their feelings of inadequacy to meet the children's needs.

Thus we came to feel that most adults do as well as they know how in their interactions with children, and would like to be able to do better, in their own eyes as well as in the opinion of others. This departure from emphasis on unrecognized (often negative) parental motives shifted the focus of need for change from the adult's emotional status to his deficits in interpersonal information, implying a very different type of intervention.

If it could be demonstrated that this change in focus could be useful, it should follow that many adults would not require clinical service, or even expert guidance, to facilitate and increase mutually satisfying interactions with their children. They might respond to experiences which provide a new, more objective, perspective: new ways of looking at interpersonal behavior which highlight characteristics that had previously been unnoticed. Through active consideration of their own interactions with children, specifically and objectively, they might identify new consequences of their own behavior for the child. In this sense, increasing adult attention to the relationship between a child's behavior and his daily interactions with parents and teachers should provide potential preventive as well as remedial benefits. In a still longer range view, techniques to facilitate objective attention to interpersonal processes could be built into schools and other socializing programs. Through these, children (the adults of the future) could learn to consider both their own social stimulus characteristics and the various means through which they too can take account of their impact on others. In effect, we were visualizing a "self-help" approach for improving human relationships. As such, goals would ultimately be educative and preventive, rather than remedial or therapeutic.

In the more immediate and pragmatic aspects of this view, there seemed to be a range of commonplace behavioral difficulties that reflect children's inability to adapt to overly complex, confusing, or contradictory interpersonal environments. These seem especially inherent in the actions of the parents and teachers upon whom children are physically and psychologically dependent. For example, unclear or inconsistent adult communications cannot evoke clear or constructive responses from the child. An experience in which the adult observes a child's confusion or anger in reaction to a contradictory adult message (e.g., by viewing a videotape wherein he smilingly berates and belittles the child) should enable many adults to identify the connection between their own behavior and the child's reaction to it. In turn, such recognition should directly define beneficial behavior changes for the adult. Further, it is hypothesized that an adult's active process of "seeing for himself" will evoke fewer avoidant and defensive reactions than having the same information suggested to him by other adults in authoritative roles, no matter how accurate and empathic such "experts" might be.

This background led to the development of an experimental intervention designed to permit adults to scan their own behavior, consider the child's daily interactional experience in relation to it, and adopt whatever changes they felt might help him. Techniques were developed for specifying and recording the objective characteristics of adult interactions with children. Graphic samples, measures, and descriptions of these interactions were collected by a relatively impersonal consultant and fed back to the involved adults under conditions that maximized attention, facilitated relatively detached and repeated scrutiny, and were as free as possible from guilt-inducing implications. Parents and teachers viewed these materials and identified the behavior they saw as injurious or provocative for the children. They could then substitute alternatives derived from their own temperamental, social, and cultural values.

Our concern to demonstrate this adult capacity and to estimate its generality and significance led to the development of the experimental intervention evaluated and described in this report. At the same time, by analyzing the children's interpersonal environment, and their reactions within it, in a variety of situations and with a number of different instruments, we hoped to gain some sense of the patterns through which child behavior and interpersonal environments are interdependent. A resulting broadened empirical base that would identify specific influences of environmental factors should in turn direct us toward a wider range of more effective remedial and preventive efforts, that is, toward new ways of reducing children's developmental difficulties.

The point of view outlined here does not minimize the importance of psychodynamic forces or the significant roles of earlier learning in the behavior of either adults or children. Nor does it deny the active and significant input of the child's own personal and temperamental characteristics into the interactional cycles. However, for a broad range of typical adjustment difficulties the realistic power of adults for determining a child's current behavior seems both a major source of difficulty and a powerful tool for change.

There is no assumption that increasing adults' information about their role in children's difficulties will solve or even ameliorate all sources of environmental stress. And it is certainly not expected to reduce significantly any of those difficulties that may be related to adult's deeply ingrained attitudes and motives. Even with these limitations, however, it seems valid to test the assumptions that *(a)* a large proportion of children's anxiety, anger, and distress stem from their conflictual and confusing interactions with parents and teachers; *(b)* through perceptual and cognitive experiences adults can come to view their interactions with children more accurately and completely; and *(c)* as a consequence of these experiences they can alter their behavior in ways that will result in demonstrable improvement in the child's functioning.

At the very least, increasing the range of professional interventions should enhance the possibility of helping those children whose parents and teachers either are *(a)* psychologically or economically unable to follow the traditional therapeutic paths of emotional self-exploration or *(b)* reject, on either overt or covert levels, directive intervention from professionals.

THEORETICAL RATIONALES FOR INFORMATION FEEDBACK

Our approach focused on the perceptions, communications, and interactions of adults with each other, and with the child, as critical variables in the adaptive* or maladaptive behavior of children. The purpose of Information Feedback procedures was to enable adults to observe interpersonal behavior and monitor their impact on children as objectively as possible. The process of providing and examining information without interpretation or evaluation by an outsider (the clinician) was expected to direct their attention to new sources of information about the relationship. Such additional information would lead to alternative perceptions and responses. In this account, we emphasize the external characteristics and effects of behavior because people's failure to recognize and monitor consequences of their behavior for others (and especially for children) is seen as a critical and largely unexplored source of interpersonal difficulty. We recognize that we present a somewhat mechanistic and incomplete segment of the total interactional process, but this seems necessary in order to explore the specific characteristics of adult behavior as a situational determinant contributing importantly to children's behavior disorders.

If we are correct in attributing some adult behavioral inadequacy to deficits in attention and information rather than to complex attitudes and motivations, the path toward remediation seems simpler. It involves providing conditions that facilitate a new way of looking at one's own and others' behavior, a perspective that extends beyond vague, habituated expectations to the identifiction of objective characteristics of behaviors that are perceived by, and have impact on, others. Since this point of view encompasses many difficulties experienced by all children in the process of learning to live adaptively with the people around them, it ultimately defines a social goal rather than a clinical problem.

There are a number of theoretical propositions that can be offered as rationales for the feedback approach. One, a perceptual model, was a major influence in the original development of the Information Feedback intervention (Kaswan, Love, & Rodnick, 1971). Briefly, this view holds that most perceptions are accurate representations of their environmental referents (Gibson, 1966). Distortions do occur, but many individual differences of-

---

* In this report we arbitrarily accept the adults' (e.g., teachers') judgments of children's desirable behavior as "adaptive."

ten regarded as distortions may represent actual differences in the stimulus characteristics to which people are responding. For example, individual perceptions vary when people attend to different aspects contained within a total stimulus range. If attention is directed to the same subsets of stimulus characteristics, through external arrangements which highlight common patterns, greater similarity in perception occurs. Thus new perceptions can be induced within familiar surroundings by incorporating previously unnoticed stimuli such as, in the interpersonal arena, examples of nonverbal behavior or tone of voice.

A second basis for individual difference in perception lies in the amount and kind of attention people direct to their environment. Practice in scanning can increase the range and specificity of attention to surroundings, increasing in turn the amount of information derived. In the interpersonal context, the identification of differences between observers as to their individual ranges and degree of detail in viewing their interaction can assist them to locate the stimulus sources of discordant percepts. The process of identifying stimulus characteristics is likely to increase the amount of overlap in people's scanning processes and in the consequent perceptions they derive.

As indicated, emphasis on the stimulus correlates of perception is considered applicable at any level of generality, including interpersonal perception. In this context, an additional source of individual variation results from the fact that the interpersonal environment is always physically different for each person. In any interaction the external visual environment for any participant includes the other but not the self; for example, no one sees himself, but only the other. Similarly, each person's voice sounds different to himself than to others because of the different distribution of sound patterns.* Thus although there is considerable overlap in the stimulus environment, there are intrinsic differences which people must learn to take into account when seeking consensus about their mutual perceptions and interactions. In bridging this particular gap, the utilization of video playback provides a unique opportunity. In this situation, each person has the novel experience of seeing himself as well as the other on the same objective plane and with the same degree of completeness. Both have access to new information that has been previously unavailable.

The point emphasized here is that perceptions, whether different from those of others or not, usually are related to objectively identifiable aspects of the environment. Although projections and distortions do occur, they do

---

* From a somewhat different perspective, Jones and Davis (1965) have also described differences in the environment experienced by actors as compared to observers in interpersonal behavior.

so under special conditions and need not be considered characteristic of the usual operation of perceptual processes. Much seemingly deviant behavior is appropriate to actual characteristics of the interpersonal environment which are unnoticed by other observers. To the extent that this is true, interpersonal behavior can be altered by changing the characteristics of the behavior that elicits it. Conversely, differences in perception can be reduced by increasing the activity, range, and specificity with which people attend to the objective characteristics of their interpersonal environment. In this sense, we are attempting to test the limits of the projective hypothesis which, in its most general form, emphasizes the idiosyncratic nature of human perceptions. It implies that each individual's perceptions are determined largely by what he is personally disposed to see, based upon his experiences, inner impulses, feelings, and fantasy. Although there is no question in our minds that such subjective mechanisms do operate, the extent to which the individual is necessarily a helpless captive of his inner life seems open to investigation. Our proposition is that many of an individual's perceptions, including person perceptions, are accurate and are realistically related to the stimuli to which he is attending. A critical corollary holds that he can increase the accuracy of his perceptions by learning to scan his total environment, adopt an objective set to attend to its characteristics, and utilize techniques through which he can verify his individual view.

Other concepts besides this perceptual model can be postulated as a basis for the Information Feedback procedures. In a Lewinian context, as described by Bennis, Schein, Steele, and Berlew (1968), the introduction of new information about an individual's interpersonal characteristics would either confirm or disconfirm his previous views of himself. Presumably confirmation would strengthen and validate the assumptions on which he had been operating whereas disconfirmation would upset expectations and set up a need for change. This is the process of "unfreezing" old patterns, of ". . . becoming open to certain kinds of information which are actually or potentially available in the environment. The process of changing is the *actual assimilation* of new information resulting in cognitive redefinition and new personal constructs. These, in turn, form the basis for new attitudes and new behavior" (p. 349). The perceptual model for Information Feedback is similar to this conception. For example, one process for achieving cognitive redefinition is scanning, the active search for information which will allow the individual to redefine his situation so as to achieve a more comfortable equilibrium. In this ". . . he relates himself primarily to the information he receives, not to the particular source from which the information comes." Changes made on this basis are described as relatively easily "refrozen" and maintained because a solution determined through the individual's own scanning is likely to fit into his personality and to be acceptable to important people around him. This scanning process is contrasted with the alternative process of "positive identification," wherein the individual uses interpersonal cues coming from a change agent with whom he identifies himself, for example, a therapist. The attempt to minimize the interpersonal influence of the clinician in Information Feedback parallels this reliance on the client's own scanning and his identification of those changes he considers desirable for himself.

From other sociopsychological points of view as well, interpersonal influence deriving from information generally is predicted to produce changes which are maintained independently of the source of the information (French & Raven, 1959; Raven, 1965). If B (in Information Feedback, the consultant) has new information which is useful to A (parent or teacher), A is likely to be influenced by the information alone, independent of B's characteristics or continued presence. From the standpoint of Kelley's attribution theory (1967), B may influence A by providing him with the means of obtaining either consistency or consensus in a new attribution. In the former case (which characterizes our Information Feedback procedures), what B provides "may consist of new analytic methods, problem-solving procedures, practice in the use of a given modality in order to increase its consistency, new perspectives and frameworks for evaluating items, training in discrimination and judgment, the suggestion of crucial comparisons in order to sharpen discriminations and evaluations, a demonstration of the relevance of facts and information that A had not previously appreciated, or instruction in relevant verbal labels. These methods have in common the property that they may be used by A independently of B. . . . The content of this influence will be adopted by and help A because it affords him attributional stability, and not because of B's expertness or credibility" (p. 201). The second method for exerting influence (persuasion) is more characteristic of Parent Counseling or Child Therapy and is more dependent on A's evaluation of B (the clinician).

Our theoretical formulation guided our questions and procedures, but in view of the scarcity of reliable empirical evidence in this field, this research is not expected to provide a critical test for any particular theory. Instead, as usual, it is hoped that our results may indicate more precise questions and potentially disconfirmable hypotheses for future studies.

THE PSYCHOSOCIAL ENVIRONMENT OF CHILDREN

Information Feedback is based on the premise that children's psychological problems are to a large extent related to difficulties in their ongoing interpersonal environment, notably the family and the school. This postulate requires evidence that the environment of children identified as disturbed differs from that of supposedly "normal" children. The collection and analysis of data relevant to this question were important objectives of this project.

The environmental emphasis represented here is shared by a number of recent conceptions of behavioral difficulties, including techniques based on theories of interpersonal communication (e.g., Watzlawick, Beavin, & Jackson, 1967), concepts of ecology as related to psychological problems (e.g., Barker, 1963; Kelly, 1966), preventive approaches like those of Caplan (1961), and community oriented applications of psychological principles (e.g., Sarason et al., 1966). All of these are based on the premise that stresses from the current environment, such as problems in communication, critically affect the probability, form, development, and outcome of adaptive and maladaptive processes. In many ways these formulations were preceded by the conceptualizations of ego psychologists like Hartman (1964, p. 15) who clearly summarized the major point of this assumption:

Adaptation is only capable of definition in relation to something else, with reference to specific environmental settings. The actual state of equilibrium achieved by a given individual tells us nothing of his capacity for adaptation so long as we have not investigated his relation with the external world.

Although the influence of environmental variables on behavior is now widely recognized, relevant empirical evidence has begun to accumulate only recently. Most of the early research on family patterns concentrated on the family context of schizophrenics. There is still relatively little that is definitely know about specific patterns of functioning which distinguish the families of nonpsychotic troubled children from those considered normal (e.g., Winter, 1971, p. 109). In recent years scattered research findings have begun to provide some indications that differences do exist in the current home environments of troubled as compared to well-functioning children (e.g., Peterson et al., 1959; Winter & Ferreira, 1969), but much of the research on this issue has yielded equivocal results (e.g., Frank, 1965). There is little evidence as to how troubled children function in relation to teachers and peers at school, and there is still less specific information about ways in which behavior at home and at school may be related to each other.

A major set of objectives for our study was to delineate interpersonal perception, communication, and interaction patterns within families of "troubled" as compared to "normal" children of elementary school age; to study the behavior of both groups of children in school; and to explore how variables in the two settings may be related in influencing the child's behavior. Consideration of differences within both groups that seemed associated with sociocultural and socioeconomic factors was an additional consistent focus.

The Family

Almost all psychological theories consider the family as somehow crucial in the psychological growth of children. In our work, the major focus was on the role of current interpersonal networks in the socialization of the child.

Many social and cultural changes are affecting family systems today, but the prime responsibility for rearing children is still assigned to the family, by both law and custom. The traditional differentiation of father and mother roles probably remains the most normatively held expectation of our culture, even though these roles too are undergoing marked and rapid changes. Insofar as the family continues to serve as a major socializing setting for the child, we view it in terms of its present, however transient, function.

Attitudes, feelings, and behavior all require identification for comparisons within and between families. Though sampling each of these, our framework led us to focus on verbal and nonverbal behavior in the communication and interaction among family members. As we use the term, effective communication refers to mutually shared understanding of verbal and nonverbal messages exchanged within a social unit. If messages are unclear, confusing, or contradictory, communication is difficult to achieve. Although people may understand each other quite well and still be in conflict, communication provides at least a common basis in terms of which conflicts potentially could be resolved. It is therefore unlikely that the family can socialize the child successfully unless its members can communicate effectively with each other, hence our emphasis on this area of familial functioning.

The School Environment

Many educators emphasize that schools play an important and active role in making children "good citizens"—in socializing them, in other words. Though this ideal remains, much has been written in recent years about the negative impact of schools on the cognitive, personal, and social development of children. Thus the schools have been accused of constricting creativity, overemphasizing conformity, and discouraging cooperative behavior. In the case of disadvantaged children, schools often have been seen as causing irreparable harm by insisting on enforcing a narrow range of social norms which are maladaptive for these children in their daily lives and which inhibit their cognitive and social growth. Many of the schools' failings have been documented amply (e.g., Silberman, 1971, pp. 53–203) and there are many proposals for educational reform. However, most research evidence refers to the outcome of content learned, as in measures of children's performance. Explanations of the interpersonal *process* which produces undesirable outcomes for children's personal and social development usually offer accumulated anecdotes as their major data. There seem to be few systematic studies of the interaction between the child and school personnel, or the relation between the child's behavior in school and at home. Since we know of no empirically testable conceptual framework delineating the components of the socialization process in school, it is not possible to be more explicit in specifying how the school environment as such, or in interaction with the home environment, may contribute to children's dysfunctional behavior. It is reasonable to consider, however, that if the children's problems are largely the result of conditions in the school, then no consistent pattern of family behaviors is likely to be associated with a child's problem identified at school. Also, if the primary determinants are situational, there may be considerable fluctuation in the behavior of children who are affected: school records and observations may indicate that they respond differently to each teacher or school setting.

METHODOLOGICAL CONSIDERATIONS

Time, money, and the availability of subjects limit the range of measures that can be used in studying children's environments. Most empirical studies of family interactions have used variations of the Strodbeck technique of stimulating family decision making (1954). Few of the reported findings have been replicated consistently and the limited situational base of much of the research makes it very difficult to relate their results to an understanding of families as complex social units (e.g., Winter, 1968). We therefore determined to sample a wider range of perceptions and behaviors in both the family and school environments. Our measures tapped four different aspects of interpersonal behavior and included data obtained from different observers and by means of different recording techniques.

All our measures were designed for dual purposes: (1) to provide data for the analysis of the child's family and school environment, and (2) to provide the content to be relayed to those parents and teachers who were assigned to the Information Feedback intervention. For the second usage, the findings from all measures were translated into distinctive, largely visual representations of salient characteristics of interpersonal behavior that could be viewed and considered by parents and teachers with a minimum of explanation or comment by the consultant.

Choice of Observational Settings

In the years since we started this study it has become fairly routine for clinicians to evaluate children's adjustment difficulties in the context of the total family system. Various theories have been postulated for the mediating effect of familial interactions on the child's present behavior patterns; these are based on a range of psychodynamic, transactional, behavior modification, and other theoretical models. However, the child's daily school experience still receives little systematic attention as a major influence on his evolving interpersonal strengths and weaknesses, with the notable exception of such programmatic work as that of Zax and Cowen (e.g., 1969). Furthermore, we know of little other normative data on the relationship between these two critical environments, home and school, in terms of their impact on the child's behavior.

Standardized contexts within which behavior can be observed are always difficult to provide. Generally, it is easier to devise situations that permit comparison of different families than it is to find a standard context for obtaining objective samples of children's interactions at school. In this investigation, all families were studied in the clinic setting; for the school data, observers went to the individual schools.

For our family measures, we included both verbal reports of behavior and samples of actual behavior within families. The need for investigation of the relationships between these two types of data has been noted often (e.g., Levinger, 1963). Two measures of each type were used. The verbal reports, obtained in the form of rating scales and questionnaires, are, as usual, incomplete representations of total behavior, lacking the significant meanings conveyed in nonverbal components. They are also subject to social desirability sets, distortions from memory defects, and the like. Similarly our behavior samples, obtained in a room with obvious observation and recording equipment, are not samples of completely natural behavior. The ethical requirement that families be aware of the public nature of their situation necessarily superseded the desire to record unconstrained interactions. Despite these limitations, we believe that our family measures tap a wide range of behaviors that are significant for an understanding of children's behavior.

School environments seem difficult to categorize. In addition to socioeconomic and cultural characteristics of pupils and teachers, there is also a unique social climate that permeates each individual school. This usually appears to reflect the philosophy and interpersonal style of the school principal. Thus each of our 10 schools represented a somewhat different type of interpersonal and social system. It would be misleading, therefore, to consider that school data collected for this study were gathered under strictly comparable conditions in the different schools. We received remarkable cooperation from most school personnel but all collaboration with our project came on top of already overburdened staff schedules. In addition, individual school staff had the usual range of ambivalent reactions to outsiders, particularly to university psychologists. As a consequence, our examination of familial interactions occurring in the clinic was more direct, detailed, and controlled than was our assessment of behavior of children, and especially of teachers, at school. Our family measures, for example, could utilize videotaped samples of adult-child interactions, but our school measures were limited to teachers' verbal reports of child behavior. We were, however, able to obtain additional systematic observations of the child's behavior in the classroom and on the playground; these were made by trained project observers.

It should be noted that the school observations do have one important advantage over the family interaction measures. They were obtained in their natural setting—the classroom and playground—whereas family interaction occurred in the relatively artificial clinic setting.

Whenever possible, we compared essentially parallel measures of parent and teacher perceptions and interactions with children, considering the role of socioeconomic factors in both.

Criteria for Sample Selection

An important requirement for a formulation encompassing both family and school influences is to consider effective as well as ineffective patterns of interaction. For this purpose, we studied the characteristics of family and school behavior of two groups of children: one who according to school personnel functioned adequately, the other made up of children who were designated by school personnel as manifesting chronic emotional problems or severe difficulty in interpersonal relationships. For the latter group, specific types of maladaptive behavior at school were identified and correlated with particular parental behavior patterns in order to determine if the child's behavior was similar at home and at school.

We selected a school sample which closely approximated the distribution of socioeconomic level and race in the Los Angeles population. In doing so, we increased the potential generalizability of results as well as the opportunity to uncover the contribution of additional variables operating in the child's family and school life.

Assessment Techniques

Our assessment focused on four aspects of interpersonal functioning. Two were verbal reports, of which one tapped interpersonal perceptions and the other elicited detailed descriptions of interpersonal behaviors. One behavior sample was designed to reflect the structural characteristics of familial communication; the other recorded both verbal and nonverbal aspects of family interaction patterns. A brief description of each of the four procedures follows.

INTERPERSONAL PERCEPTIONS

The evaluative views that parents, children, and teachers have of themselves and each other were sampled, as was the degree to which each person was aware of how others regarded him. To obtain this information, we developed an Adjective Rating Scale to be used as a standard reference framework within the project. The adjectives (e.g., rude, friendly, bored) provided a means for getting comparable ratings of people and interpersonal behavior in several situations (family, school, clinic) by different people (parents, teachers, children, project raters). Consistent use of the same adjectives permitted identification of relationships in perceived behavior (both consistencies and differences) in different situations and interpersonal contexts, and in the viewpoints of different observers.

The process of making these ratings required the individual's consideration of the terms in which people perceive each other, thus directing attention to the interpersonal arena. For the purposes of the Information Feedback intervention, sets of these ratings were drawn up as colored graphs on transparent sheets. These, superimposed to permit direct comparisons, were shown to parents and teachers for study and discussion in their feedback sessions.

DESCRIPTIONS OF INTERPERSONAL BEHAVIOR

The specific characteristics of the behavior of children and adults were elicited through an extensive questionnaire filled out by parents and teachers. Questions included types and frequencies of behavior, the contexts within which they occur, their antecedents, and their consequences. The concrete formulation of the questions required detailed reflection about current behaviors and their immediate consequences. Parent and teacher responses were examined and shared in feedback sessions.

CHARACTERISTICS OF VERBAL COMMUNICATION IN FAMILIES

Characteristics of the verbal communication used by parents and children were explored in a Family Communication Task which sampled the interchanges of parents and child in a standardized information exchange situation. This task was designed to explore accuracy of verbal messages in families and the processes through which information is given and sought. The findings within each family were again part of the material considered in Information Feedback sessions.

PATTERNS OF FAMILY BEHAVIOR

The type, frequency, and scope of behaviors among family members were investigated by each of the three means of inquiry just described: evaluative ratings, behavioral reports, and analysis of verbal communication. Another major source of information about observable family behavior was obtained by videotaping each family in a standardized setting during the initial 15–20 minutes of their first appointment in the clinic. (Families had always received a letter describing the recording procedures used in the clinic before coming for their first visit and had had opportunities to raise questions or concerns about observation and/or recordings.)

Although the public nature of the situation was evident to the family, the recorded behaviors seem to be valid examples of family interaction. Other researchers have demonstrated that the fact of being observed does not completely inhibit significant characteristics of interaction (e.g., Schulman, Shoemaker, and Moelis, 1962). It has also been noted that in such observed situations *process* is more difficult to mask than *content* (Levinger, 1963). On this basis we expected that although the things people would do and say in these interactions would be altered sharply relative to their behavior in natural settings, the *way* in which they behaved should still be continuous with their personal styles and interpersonal patterns. Verbalizations might be selectively censored but style of talking, nonverbal posture, physical proximity, eye contact, and a host of other indicators should be less subject to voluntary alteration and control.

We similarly expected that the recorded interactions would be altered in a positive direction so as to appear "nicer" than real life patterns would reflect. Lennard and Bernstein (1969) have noted that concordance or harmonious relationships occur less in families than other social groups. "It appears that the family context (studied in a laboratory setting) generates more discordance and disagreement than do *ad hoc* laboratory groups or other special purpose systems such as psychotherapy. One would suspect that the ratio of concordance might be still lower in 'natural' family interaction" (p. 90).

The videotapes provide permanent records of family behavior and permit the detailed and repeated scrutiny necessary for complex analyses. For example, these tapes made it feasible to study both verbal and nonverbal aspects of family communication in detail, as reported in Chapter 4. Viewing and rating their videotapes by family members also formed an important part of the Information Feedback intervention.

Basic Dimensions for the Analysis of Interpersonal Behavior

Though they vary greatly in type, our four ways of characterizing behavior all deal with interpersonal phenomena. To provide a consistent framework reflecting the connotative content of these diverse data, we adopted a modification of Osgood's well-known dimensions: evaluation, potency, and activity (Osgood, Suci, & Tannenbaum, 1957). These three have been found to account for a good deal of the variance of affective meanings in both verbal and nonverbal domains (Osgood, 1962). Versions of the evaluative and potency dimensions also appear as major axes in most attempts to conceptualize general dimensions of interpersonal behavior (e.g., Leary, 1957; Schutz, 1958). In terms of parental behavior, factor analyses have identified two commonly agreed upon dimensions which may be considered variations of evaluation and potency: acceptance versus rejection, and permissiveness versus restrictive control (Becker, 1964). In view of this general agreement, there was reason to believe that a version of Osgood's dimensions would tap basic aspects of behavior, account for a substantial amount of the variance in behavior ratings, and provide a unifying frame of reference for findings from our diverse measures. Accordingly, positive or negative evaluative characteristics, active or inactive behavioral stances, and differing types of interpersonal influence efforts manifested in family and school settings are considered throughout the study.

Guidelines for Data Analysis

For the most part, results of all measures were analyzed with mixed design analysis of variance procedures (Hays, 1963, p. 439). None of our measures satisfied strict interval or ratio scale demands, but care was taken to convert scales to standard scores or use other transformations where necessary to reduce heterogeneity of variance. Under these circumstances, the power and flexibility of analysis of variance techniques seem justified if results are interpreted with caution. Where the measures contained many scales or items, as in the Adjective Rating Scale or Behavior Inventory, we factor-analyzed the scales, using Kaiser Varimax orthogonal rotations and taking care to replicate factor structures with pilot groups. For our present purposes, we had little interest in the factor structure of the instruments as such, but rather sought to obtain groupings of items so that comparisons between groups on different sets of items within an instrument would have minimal correlation among the sets.

With our large pool of data a great number of comparisons could be made, so that there is substantial probability that the statistical significance of individual comparisons is due to chance. To help guard against this danger individual comparisons, even if they approach customary levels of statistical significance, usually are not discussed unless they are replicated or otherwise supported (e.g., in different measures, by different observers, or in different situations). Throughout, we tried to offer interpretations predominantly on the basis of converging evidence. Means and statistical tests are reported only where the results can be presented simply. In most of the chapters, where there are many and complex results, the direction of differences is reported only where the probability level of comparisons exceeded $p < .10$. Appendix B provides the statistical details for these chapters.

CHAPTER 2

The Study Population

The study involved 10 schools and 120 families. They were chosen from areas representing the range of socioeconomic levels within the West Elementary District of the Los Angeles City School System. According to Hollingshead's (1958) criterion of socioeconomic level (SEL), three schools were in upper-middle-class (Hi) areas; four were in middle-class (Mid) areas; and three were in mid to upper levels of lower (Lo) socioeconomic levels. Details as to the identification of families and schools in terms of SEL are provided in Appendix A, p. 232.

Of the participating families, 91 had a child considered by school personnel as having chronic and severe adjustment problems. When parents concurred, they were referred to the UCLA Psychology Department Clinic for psychological help for the child's problems. The other 29 families in the study, termed nonreferred (NR), contained a child who had been selected by school personnel as matching a referred (R) child in age, sex, general intelligence, ethnic origin, socioeconomic level, and classroom teacher. Because our design required a comparison among three methods of clinical intervention, a relatively large number of referred children was needed to provide samples adequate for statistical comparison among the three treatment groups. Our budget did not permit selection of both a large treatment group and a "normal" control group of equal size. Our planned solution to this problem was to match 30 nonreferred children to a random sample of one-third of the projected 90 "disturbed" children on ecological (classroom, school) and demographic variables. The controls would thus be as representative as possible of the referred group for all variables except the adequacy of the child's interpersonal behavior and, of course, the associated differences in the motivation of the two groups of families in coming to the clinic. All control families were offered professional feedback about themselves as the incentive for their participation in the study. On this basis a matched sample of NR families was obtained for all but one of the randomly identified 30 referred children.

Our goal was to sample a broad spectrum of families with children manifesting emotional and behavioral difficulties in elementary schools. We were, of course, limited to families in which parents were themselves concerned about their child's problem, and who would seek assistance at a university facility. Although there was some curtailment of cases at both extremes of the socioeconomic range, our sample seems generally representative of families with children exhibiting serious interpersonal difficulties in Los Angeles elementary schools.

The selection of schools on the basis of SEL differentiation, however, resulted in automatic ethnic separation as well. The 64 referred caucasian families were all in the Hi and Mid SEL levels; the 22 black cases were all Lo SEL. In addition, the latter group included one Mexican-American, one Oriental, and one Polynesian family, plus two families in which the father was black and the mother white. Though we had planned to study both SEL and ethnic characteristics in child and family comparisons, in view of the ethnic-SEL overlap our analyses and interpretations were restricted to SEL groupings.

Table 1 presents the characteristics of our study population with respect to some of the variables on which child and family differences might be reflected. Percentages or group means in the table permit comparisons between referred and nonreferred families and between families at high, middle, and low socioeconomic levels. Individual entries in Table 1 are discussed in the text when they show statistically significant differences ($p <$ .05) or strong trends ($p < .1$) between R/NR or SEL criterion groups. The relationship of these variables with the child's predominant type of difficulty (referral category) is presented later in this chapter.

REFERRED—NONREFERRED AND SOCIOECONOMIC LEVEL COMPARISONS

Family Composition

R/NR COMPARISONS

Staff in participating schools had indicated from the outset that it would not be possible to match nonreferred to referred children on the basis of family composition. Table 1 shows that in fact *twice as many referred children (48% as compared to 24%) came from homes containing either a single parent or a stepparent.* This finding is in line with the high incidence of broken homes that has long been noted in families of children with behavioral disturbances (e.g., Glueck & Glueck, 1950).

Of the 91 referred families, 29 contained only one parent. Single-parent families thus made up 32% of the referred group. Of these the father was absent in 25 homes; four other families had no mother. For nonreferred

Table 1. Sample Characteristics

N	Referred (91)		Nonreferred (29)		Socioeconomic Level: R + NR					
					Hi (27)		Mid (60)		Lo (33)	
Socioeconomic level										
Hi	21	(.23)	6	(.21)						
Mid	45	(.50)	15	(.51)						
Lo	25	(.27)	8	(.28)						
Family Composition N (%)										
Single parent	29	(.32)	2	(.07)	3	(.11)	11	(.17)	17	(.52)
Stepparent	15	(.16)	5	(.17)	5	(.19)	13	(.22)	3	(.09)
Both natural parents	47	(.52)	22	(.76)	19	(.70)	36	(.61)	13	(.39)
Number of family moves (Mean)	3.70		2.46		2.09		3.45		4.24	
FRPV IQ (Mean)										
Child	116.7		124.3		130.8		120.0		107.6	
Father	108.8		108.9		116.1		109.1		94.1	
Mother	100.9		108.5		111.4		105.3		92.2	

Age (Mean)					
Child	9.4	9.5	9.0	9.6	9.6
Father	39.6[a]	39.0[c]	40.7	39.8	36.8
Mother	35.4[b]	36.9[d]	37.2	36.6	33.4
Sex of Child N (%)					
Male	74 (.81)	25 (.86)	23 (.85)	46 (.76)	30 (.91)
Female	17 (.19)	4 (.14)	4 (.15)	14 (.24)	3 (.09)
Grades (Mean)					
Academic	2.39	2.94	2.51	2.15	1.83
Physical education	2.05	3.26	2.73	2.46	2.30
Music-art	2.63	3.11	2.51	2.47	2.17
Conduct	2.43	2.81	2.32	1.99	1.56
Birth Order					
Only child	14 (.15)	3 (.10)	3 (.11)	9 (.15)	5 (.15)
Oldest	36 (.40)	8 (.28)	10 (.37)	21 (.35)	13 (.40)
Younger	41 (.45)	18 (.52)	14 (.52)	31 (.50)	15 (.45)
Number of Children (Mean)	2.47	2.62	2.56	2.38	2.70

[a] $N=69$.   [b] $N=86$.   [c] $N=27$.   [d] $N=29$.

23

families only two homes were without a father (7%) and all contained a mother. Thus as school personnel had predicted, the two sets of families proved to be very different in terms of parental composition, with much higher levels of disruption appearing in families of children with social adjustment problems. Adopted children, however, were represented similarly in both groups (6% of the referred, 3% of the nonreferred).

SEL COMPARISONS

Family composition also varied in relation to socioeconomic level. For the total sample of 120 families, including both referred and nonreferred, Lo SEL families were significantly higher than the other SEL groups in the incidence of broken homes. *For all kinds of disruption (single-parent, stepparent, and adoptive homes), the percentage of Lo SEL families was almost twice that of the Mid and Hi SEL groups (61% in comparison with 39% and 30%, respectively).*

When only single-parent homes are considered, 52% of Lo SEL families were represented, whereas both Mid and Hi SELs had less than 20% in this category. This difference is significant at $p < .01$. The percentage of single-parent families in the total sample (26%) is just double the 13% estimate of American children being raised in one-parent families cited in the Final Report of the Joint Commission on the Mental Health of Children (1970, p. 23). The reputation of the Southern California urban area for high levels of familial disruption seems indeed to be justified, with highest incidence being clearly related to low socioeconomic conditions.

Within the low socioeconomic level, the one-parent and stepparent families were concentrated in the Lo SEL *referred* subgroup; Lo SEL nonreferred families were as likely to have both natural parents living in the home as were Hi or Mid SEL controls.

Finally, in the referred, Lo SEL, single-parent homes, the missing parent was always the father. Table 2 presents the relationships of type of father (natural or step) in the home with SEL.

Thus our data support the usual expectation that the presence of both natural parents in the home seems associated with higher likelihood of the child's good adjustment at school. The absence of the father seems more

Table 2.   Fathers in Referred Families as Related to Socioeconomic Level

N	Hi (21)		Mid (45)		Lo (25)	
Natural father	14	(67%)	25	(63%)	8	(32%)
Stepfather	4	(19%)	10	(17%)	2	(8%)
No father	3	(14%)	7	(19%)	15	(60%)

characteristic of poor school adjustment for Lo SEL than higher SEL children (though other factors associated with the Lo SEL child's difficulties will be reported later).

Family Mobility: Number of Moves in the Last 10 Years

R/NR COMPARISONS

The referred families were somewhat more mobile in their living patterns than the nonreferreds but the differences were only a trend ($t = 1.8$, $p <$ .1). There was much more variation in mobility within the nonreferred than the referred group. A committee report from the 1970 White House Conference on Children emphasized the disruptive effect of family moves for grade-school children (Epstein, 1971, p. 5), but our data in Table 1 indicate that increased family mobility is not strongly associated with psychological disturbance per se. Instead, the *family moves seem more related to socioeconomic level, with Hi SEL the least mobile and Lo SEL the most* (p < .05). Our Hi SEL families tended to be professionally well established; the Mid SEL were often upward-mobile; the Lo SEL were usually transient, making more moves, presumably to seek economic opportunities. These mobility trends were parallel for referred and nonreferred families and follow the pattern indicated in the 1970 Joint Commission Report: one-fifth of all American families move each year and this mobility is "particularly high among very young, non-white, and low-income families" (p. 23).

Full Range Picture-Vocabulary (FRPV) IQ

This test was used as a rough screening for functional verbal facility relevant to our project tasks. Information about this test and our administration and use of it is presented in Appendix A, p. 232. The children's scores reported in Table 1 appear to reflect inflated estimates of intelligence as usually measured. Scores obtained by mothers and fathers seem more compatible with usual group estimates of adult verbal intelligence.

R/NR COMPARISONS

Comparisons of mean IQ on this picture-vocabulary test indicate that control families gained somewhat higher scores than did referred families. The relationship between membership in the R versus NR groups for different family members was evaluated through an overall Group (R, NR) × Family Members (father, mother, child) analysis of variance. This yielded a group effect (NR/R) significant at $p < .05$. Differences in terms of the different family members, however, were significant only for comparisons between referred and nonreferred mothers' scores. *Our matching of children therefore seems to have resulted in child and father groups with roughly equivalent intellectual, or at least verbal, capacity.*

SEL COMPARISONS

Socioeconomic level analyses based on the total sample of 120 families showed that IQ as measured here was positively related to SEL for all family members. SEL Group × Members (Fa, Mo, Ch) × R/NR analyses of variance yielded highly significant main group effects ($p < .001$). There was a very clear association of socioeconomic level with IQ indices in all families, control as well as referred. As Table 1 shows, this effect is not due simply to differences between extreme groups, but to a consistent decrease in IQ scores from Hi to Mid to Lo, in that order.

The better educational background of Hi SEL parents may well have enriched their vocabulary and made it possible for them to provide a more stimulating verbal environment for their children. But this explanation of the SEL finding would imply that the difference between Hi and Mid SEL groups with respect to verbal and educational levels is as great as that between Mid and Lo—a concept not often posited. Certainly, the factors of sociocultural deprivation or ethnic background often invoked to explain poor IQ scores of Lo SEL groups do not seem applicable to the Mid SEL families. Other indications of this linear relationship occur and are discussed further, in the context of other data.

Possible R/NR differences in FRPV IQ scores were analyzed for individual family members within each SEL level (see Appendix B, Table 1). The only statistically significant finding was that nonreferred Mid SEL mothers and children scored significantly higher on this test than did Mid SEL referred mothers and children. A possible interpretation of this result is offered in the context of the predominant behavior problems of Mid SEL children which are discussed in the final section of this chapter.

Age of Child

Since age of the child was one of the matching criteria for control children, there were no R/NR differences on this variable.

In SEL comparisons, the ages of our children at referral did not support the findings of McDermott, Harrison, Schrager, and Wilson (1965) that lower-class children are referred for professional help at older ages than children of fathers in "skilled" occupations. The role of school personnel in initiating referral in our study may well be reflected here. Their opportunity to refer Lo SEL children for treatment at low, or no, fee may have resulted in identification of problem behaviors at earlier ages than would have occurred otherwise.

Age of Parents

Table 1 indicates that parents of Lo SEL children tended to be younger than the parents of other children, but this effect is not statistically significant ($p < .10$). The absence of the natural father in 68% of Lo SEL referred homes makes it difficult to compare our parental ages with data gathered from Lo SEL two-parent families. One study (Speer et al., 1968) investigated a sample of original two-parent families who attended at least three appointments in a psychiatric child guidance clinic. These lower-class fathers were much older than their wives and were also older than the middle-class fathers in the same sample. The selection criteria employed in that study would yield a sample with much higher levels of family stability than our criteria produced.

Sex of Child

The four to one male-female ratio for our referred sample is in the range generally reported for referrals of children of elementary school age (e.g., Hunt, 1962). The sex ratio in the control group is the same, of course, since sex was one of the matching criteria.

Mid SEL schools referred the most girls for psychological treatment and Lo SEL schools the fewest, but the proportion of male-female referrals was not statistically different for the three SEL groups.

School Grades

Children's school grades were used in several ways in this study. Details of the numerical conversions and factor analyses made of grades are presented in Appendix A, pp. 233-234. These provided four separate grade groupings for each child: his scores for music-art, physical education, conduct, and academic subjects, as indicated in Table 1.

R/NR COMPARISONS

Grades awarded for all types of school subjects and activities are intimately associated with the perceived adequacy of children's behavioral adjustment at school, according to our data. Results of a Group (R, NR) $\times$ Grade Category analysis of variance with an F at $p < .001$ indicate substantial R $<$ NR differences. Separate analyses were made on each of the four grade factors, academic, physical education, music-art, and conduct; R/NR differences were significant ($p < .01$) for each grouping of grades. Since disturbed children usually do less well in school than relatively untroubled youngsters (e.g., Crandall et al., 1964), this finding is to be expected. It is interesting to observe that the greatest R/NR difference appears in the physical education scores.

SEL COMPARISONS

SEL analyses indicate that there are also significant relationships between a child's socioeconomic background and his school grades. These relationships were studied by a SEL × (R, NR) × Grade analysis of variance yielding a SEL group F at $p < .01$. Individual t tests between SEL levels in each grade category were also computed. *The Hi SEL group received the highest grades; Mid SEL received lower grades; and Lo SEL received lowest grades, in all categories.* It is possible that this finding reflects different teacher orientations toward the various socioeconomic groups. For example, Leacock (1969) and others have emphasized that middle-class teachers convey an image for lower-class children "which expects deviance to be unruliness with regard to behavior and apathy with regard to curriculum" (p. 181). In the absence of data, however, the simplest explanation is that this grade-SEL relationship may merely reflect the IQ distribution (functional verbal facility) which it parallels.

Socioeconomic level effects on grades were manifested differently in the referred and nonreferred groups. (The analysis of variance yielded significant interactions between R/NR and SEL at $p < .01$. These are shown in Figure 1.) *Both Hi and Mid SEL groups reflected distinct differences between referred and nonreferred children in all grade categories. All Lo SEL children, however, received about the same low grades in academic and cultural subjects whether they were seen as troubled (R) or not (NR).* R/NR differentiation for these children was reflected only for physical education and conduct grades. It would appear that inferior physical development and motor coordination and/or socialization with respect to group membership and adult authority (e.g., following orders) were critical determinants leading to referral of Lo SEL children. Since physical education grades had reflected the largest R/NR differences for the total group as well, the possible significance of physical education grades may merit further investigation.

Birth Order

R/NR COMPARISONS

There were no clear differences between referred and nonreferred groups with respect to birth order in these data. Some studies in social psychology in recent years have suggested that "only" and oldest children are more likely to have interpersonal difficulty than those born later into the family (e.g., Schachter, 1959; Warren, 1966). The trend shown in Table 1 is consonant with this assumption but is not statistically significant (chi square, $p <$

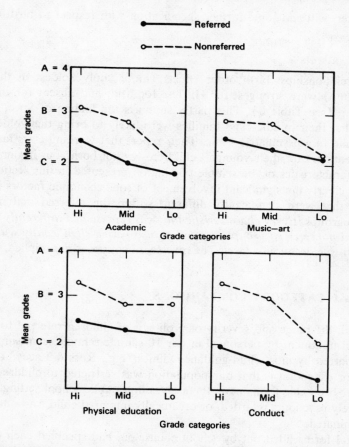

Figure 1. Grades as related to socioeconomic level and referred-nonreferred groupings.

.11). *Within* the referred group, however, there was a significant birth order effect: here the group containing "only" and oldest children received *better* academic and conduct grades than children who came later in the family sequence. As noted, Table 1 shows that referred children in general received worse grades than the nonreferred, and this seems to be the usual expectation. If "only"/oldest children are more troubled than their younger siblings, they might be expected to receive *poorer* grades, even within the referred group. Although our finding might be related to some other factor such as the higher achievement motivation often attributed to the older child, we have no data to help resolve this point. Differentiations within the referred group in terms of different types of problems, presented later in this chapter, will add some further specification with respect to birth order effects.

SEL COMPARISONS

In SEL relationships, birth order effects (more "only"/oldest in the referred group) were strongest for Hi, less for Mid, and absent for the Lo SEL group (see Table 3). This partly supports the finding of Speer et al (1968) that their middle-class families were likely to bring their oldest or "only" child to a psychiatric clinic. Their report that working-class families sought treatment for their youngest children was not borne out in our data.

The characteristics of the sample population presented in this section reflect very clearly the significant involvement of socioeconomic factors in the variables that were significantly different within the referred and nonreferred subgroups. *Every characteristic that was represented differently in referred and nonreferred groups of families also varied significantly with differences in socioeconomic level.* The reverse, of course, is not implied.

REFERRAL CATEGORY COMPARISONS

In general, the range and severity of problems of children referred for psychological treatment by personnel in our 10 sample schools seem similar to those reported by most child-guidance clinics (e.g., Ross & Lacey, 1961). The major exception is that our population was restricted to children who had so far been able to maintain themselves in a public-school setting. Thus the severely psychotic, retarded, or organically impaired child was automatically eliminated.

Referral forms filled out by school counselors had specified each child's behavioral and emotional difficulties. These statements were weighted and classified into four categories. (1) Aggressiveness (Ag): the child expresses anger physically, is hostile, disruptive, and uncooperative, and defies authority. (2) Hyperactivity (Hy): the child is restless, shows compulsive moving and/or talking, and has poor peer relationships. (3) Social Withdrawal

Table 3.   Birth Order Percentages: SEL and R/NR Comparisons

Birth Order	Hi		Mid		Lo	
	R	NR	R	NR	R	NR
Only	10	17	16	13	20	0
Oldest	52	17	36	20	36	50
Younger	38	66	48	67	44	50

(SW): the child is anxious, insecure, low in self-confidence, and dependent on teacher. (4) Poor Attention Control (AC): he manifests poor work habits, immaturity, and distractibility. Details of the procedures for constructing the categories and assigning children to them are found in Appendix A, pp. 234-236.

The characteristics of the referred children's adjustment difficulties were studied in two ways: (1) by the prevalence and severity of the four types of disturbed behavior in the total sample; and (2) by the incidence of children who showed each type of disturbance as their predominant difficulty.

Seriousness Attributed to the Four Types of Problem Behaviors in the Referred Sample

Sorting the items from all referral statements for all referred children into the four categories showed the prevalence and severity that school personnel attributed to the four problem behaviors as such. Table 4 gives the mean severity scores for the four problem behaviors when the referral statements for

Table 4.   Analysis in Terms of Teacher Reports of Problem Behaviors: Mean Severity Scores for Individual Referral Categories

	Aggression	Hyper-activity	Social Withdrawal	Attention Control	Total Severity Index
$N=91$	2.60	2.44	3.47	4.34	
SEL					
Hi	2.78	2.77	3.39	4.59	6.54
Mid	1.96	2.21	4.22	4.36	6.73
Lo	3.50	2.49	2.05	3.93	6.46
Family composition					
Single parent	2.81	2.68	2.32	5.13	6.50
Stepparent	1.68	2.55	4.05	4.12	6.44
Both natural parents	2.73	2.18	3.92	4.24	6.70
Sex					
Male	2.75	2.61	3.38	4.53	6.62
Female	1.95	1.71	3.88	3.54	6.53
Birth order					
Only	1.69	2.17	3.91	4.62	6.60
Oldest	1.99	2.56	3.69	4.29	6.66
Younger	3.35	2.41	3.14	4.30	6.56

the 91 referred cases were grouped for various analyses. Statements about Hyperactivity occurred least often and with least severe implications; this disturbance therefore appeared lowest in severity of the four. Poor Attention Control was the highest (mentioned most often and described as most severe). Involving children in task oriented classwork is typically foremost among teacher's concerns, so that emphasis on this category is not surprising in a classification based on children's behavior in school. Social Withdrawal was second highest in severity as an overall problem. This finding would tend to refute the usual notion that teachers do not perceive quiet, shy children as psychologically troubled. These teachers apparently identified social inhibition as a deficit in children's optimal functioning and did not value it as desirable conformity or malleability in the classroom.

Severity scores for the four referral categories differed with respect to the three socioeconomic levels. A Referral Category × SEL analysis of variance of the sample means in Table 4 yielded a significant Referral Category effect ($p < .05$) and a SEL × Referral Category interaction ($p < .05$). For all three SEL groups, Attention Control problems were highest, again reflecting the situational basis of the identification process. *Teachers in Hi and Lo SEL schools reported more severe problems with aggressive and hyperactive behavior than did those in Mid SEL, whereas teachers in Mid SEL schools characteristically described Social Withdrawal as the predominant symptom.* Overall, Mid SEL reports varied over the widest range of severity for the different types of problems. Within referral categories, Social Withdrawal had more SEL variation than any other, with highest scores for Mid and lowest for Lo SEL.

Except for this SEL variation there seemed to be little relationship between referral category and the other seven variables, e.g., family composition, reported earlier in this chapter. [This was determined through Pearson r correlations computed between severity scores and other variables in the sample whenever *(a)* the sample variable had a continuous score and *(b)* the sample variance of the two distributions was reasonably similar. Only two significant correlations emerged; since these could well have resulted from chance, and have no substantiation in other data, they are not reported.]

Classification of Children According to their Predominant Problem

The second analysis of referral problems was based on the categorization of each child in terms of his predominant difficulty. Though a child's referral statement often contained items that fell into two or more categories, for purposes of this analysis he was classified under the one on which he manifested greatest incidence and severity, that is, had the highest severity score. The number of cases in each of the four referral categories shown in Table 5 indicates an almost equal number of cases with predominantly Aggressive

Table 5. Classification of Children by Predominant Referral Category

	Aggression (N = 22)			Hyperactivity (N = 15)			Social Withdrawal (N = 18)			Attention Control (N = 35)		
	N	%	a	N	%	a	N	%	a	N	%	a
SEL												
Hi	6	.29	5.73	4	.24	5.67	3	.14	6.08	8	.33	5.78
Mid	7	.16	6.41	5	.11	4.72	13	.30	6.98	20	.44	6.40
Lo	9	.36	6.18	6	.24	5.53	2	.08	4.95	8	.32	6.33
Family Composition												
One parent	9	.31	5.52	7	.24	5.47	2	.07	8.79	11	.38	6.15
Stepparent	2	.13	6.17	2	.13	3.65	6	.38	6.25	6	.38	6.01
Both natural parents	13	.28	6.28	6	.13	5.97	10	.22	6.37	17	.37	6.39
Sex												
Male	17	.23	6.63	14	.19	6.20	13	.18	6.58	29	.41	6.84
Female	5	.29	7.28	1	.06	6.86	6	.35	6.40	5	.29	5.75
Birth order												
Only	1		7.05	1		4.00	6		7.31	6		5.56
Oldest	8		6.19	7		5.48	7		6.65	14		6.11
Younger	13		6.10	8		5.38	5		5.68	15		6.66
Total severity scores			6.77			6.25			6.58			5.90
Grades (X)												
Academic			1.93			2.00			2.26			1.87
Physical education			2.48			2.31			2.39			2.24
Music-art			2.24			2.38			2.44			2.28
Conduct			1.56			1.69			2.17			1.47

[a] Mean Severity Scores for children *including* scores on secondary categories.

(N = 22), Hyperactive (N = 16), and Social Withdrawal (N = 18) problems. The Attention Control category, with 35 children, clearly had more cases than any of the other three, again probably reflecting the teacher's concern with task orientation. The items in this category also were mentioned most often, so that Attention Control severity scores are typically larger than scores for other referral categories.

The SEL comparisons in Table 5 show that Mid SEL children's referral category pattern was different from both Hi and Lo SEL in their high scores for Social Withdrawal and low scores for Hyperactivity. When Mid SEL children are disturbed, they apparently tend to evidence their difficulties in personal inhibition, in contrast to Hi and Lo SEL children who give more overt interpersonal expression to their disturbance. A chi square for the whole table was not significant, however.

Analyses of both types of classification—the seriousness attributed to the four types of problem behavior in the total sample and the classification of children according to their predominant type of disturbance—led to similar results with respect to SEL: *both reflected a high incidence of inhibited behavior in Mid SEL children, and of inadequately restrained behavior in both Hi and Lo SEL groups.*

Besides the SEL comparisons just described, two other variables were significantly related to the children's predominant type of problem: school grades and birth order.

Children manifesting different types of difficulties differed somewhat on school grades (see Table 5). A Grades × Referral Category analysis of variance (mean grades of children in each referral category) was significant at $p < .05$. Attention Control children with their problems of task orientation tended to have the worst grades whereas Social Withdrawal children had the best. It should be noted, however, that the single highest mean grade was 2.48, a C+ obtained by aggressive children in physical education. Thus the relatively better grades of the SW children are at such a low level they cannot be taken as an indication that the children's poor social interaction was a consequence of absorption in a superior learning process.

The other referral category relationship indicated in our data is with birth order. Earlier in this chapter it was reported that there was a trend for "only"/oldest children to appear more commonly in referred than nonreferred families ($p < .11$). A separate analysis of referral categories reveals that *"only"/oldest children appear significantly more often in the Social Withdrawal category than would be expected from the birth order relationships within our control children* (Appendix B, Table 2). *Furthermore, the tendency for "only" and oldest children to manifest socially inhibited behavior holds particularly for Mid SEL children* (Appendix B, Table 3).

The birth order effect sometimes has been seen as possibly related to closeness to the mother (the maternal overprotection syndrome, e.g., Levy, 1943). From this point of view the tendency of Mid SEL children to manifest problems of inhibition and fearfulness suggests a possible relationship with the lower IQ levels achieved by these children and their mother relative to the Mid SEL control group. The IQ index was obtained through a picture-vocabulary task administered in an interpersonal situation. If these children were modeling their behavior after their mothers (in a stereotyped middle class, retiring interpersonal style), performance of both referred mothers and children might well suffer on a recognition task administered by a strange person in a somewhat formidable setting. Situational constraints might reduce their spontaneous verbalization, restrict their use of guesses, and the like. A similar process of high discomfort in a strange setting may also account for some of the poor performance of the Lo SEL group in this task. These possibilities are, of course, entirely speculative.

Three general conclusions seem warranted by the group comparisons reported thus far:

1. *With respect to the family and school variables examined here, the total sample seems generally representative of a broad spectrum of the elementary school children in the Los Angeles area.*

2. *The matching procedures for control cases seem to have been reasonably successful in providing referred and nonreferred groups that are similar with respect to background variables.*

3. *Results highlight the interrelationship of familial, socioeconomic, and sociocultural factors with the child's adaptive functioning in urban public school settings. The need for explicit consideration of familial and SEL factors in all estimates of children's functioning is underlined in these results.*

PART ONE

Families and Schools

CHAPTER 3

The Child in the Family: Verbal Reports

Information about the child and his family was obtained by means of four techniques which focused on the patterns of interpersonal evaluation, activity, and efforts at interpersonal influence that were demonstrated within the families. Findings from each instrument will be presented in turn and then discussed together. More detail about the statistical background and treatment of each instrument is available in Appendix A.

The two techniques based on verbal reports are ratings by family members on the Family Adjective Rating Scales (FARS) and inventories of family behaviors as described by parents (Parent Behavior Inventory, PBI). Results of the two techniques which sampled behavior—responses to a Family Communication Task, and videotapes of family interactions during a standardized sequence of conditions—are presented in the next chapter.

Of the four techniques, the videotapes were planned for all families. Because of design considerations associated with the treatment comparisons (see Chapter 7), the FARS, PBI, and Family Communication Task were projected for all NR families and those receiving Information Feedback, but for only half the families in the Child Therapy and Parent Counseling interventions.

FAMILY ADJECTIVE RATING SCALE

The scale contained 10 adjectives representing interpersonal attributes and behavior. Each rater judged the extent (never to always) to which each adjective characterized himself and other members of the family. In order to provide a more uniform rating context and thus improve the reliability and validity of the scales, every rater was presented with a set of standard definitions of the adjectives. To ensure that all project participants would have a comparable understanding of the words (including children as young as 8 years old and adults with minimal education), the definitions used were collected from fourth, fifth, and sixth graders in a ghetto school outside the project area. The adjectives and their definitions were as follows.

1. *Active.* Active means doing a lot of things and being busy.
2. *Bored.* Bored means having nothing to do or being tired of what's going on.
3. *Patient.* Patient means being willing to wait.
4. *Rude.* Rude means being impolite.
5. *Afraid.* Afraid means being scared.
6. *Controlling.* Controlling means getting others to do something.
7. *Phony.* Phony means putting on an act.
8. *Friendly.* Friendly means liking other people and being nice to them.
9. *Angry.* Angry means being mad.
10. *Clear.* Clear means what is being said is easy to understand.

In addition to the denotative anchors provided by the definitions, connotative meanings were assessed routinely through Semantic Differential techniques, each rater evaluating each adjective separately for its evaluative, activity, and potency dimensions. The results of the semantic ratings indicated almost universal agreement on the connotations of the words. It was tenable, therefore, to assume that the adjectives had highly similar connotative meanings for the individual raters. Tests of the validity of the adjectives for distinguishing between a variety of psychologically troubled and nontroubled populations are reported in Appendix A, pp. 236-242.

Ratings discussed in this chapter were obtained during the families' first visit to the clinic. After having rated each adjective on the Semantic Differential scales, fathers, mothers, and target children (referred or control) used the 10 adjectives to rate six concepts. Each adjective was marked along a nine point scale ranging from "never" to "always," for how often it applied to the concept person or situation. Parents rated the concepts: *myself, my spouse, my child, how my spouse will rate me, how my child will rate me,* and *the average person of my age and sex.* The child rated: *myself, my mother, my father, how my mother will rate me, how my father will rate me,* and *how I rate my teacher.* A sample sheet (Figure 2) shows the concept to be rated, with the 10 adjectives and their "never" to "always" scale below.

The father and mother did their ratings simultaneously, seated at tables at opposite sides of one room. The child's ratings were obtained concurrently in another room. Project workers were present in both situations to provide clarification and assistance as needed, but uniformity of presentation for adult raters was ensured by having the adjectives presented over a tape recorder. The tape presented an adjective with its standard definition and allowed 7 seconds for the rater to record his evaluation. In occasional instances where parents could not proceed at this pace, the adjectives were

Date ____

Do not write in this space

0 1 2 3 4 5 6 7 8 9   0 1 2 3 4 5 6 7 8 9

HOW MY MOTHER WILL RATE ME

Rater ____ (Child)

Bored	Not at all		Very much
Patient	Not at all		Very much
Afraid	Not at all		Very much
Controlling	Not at all		Very much

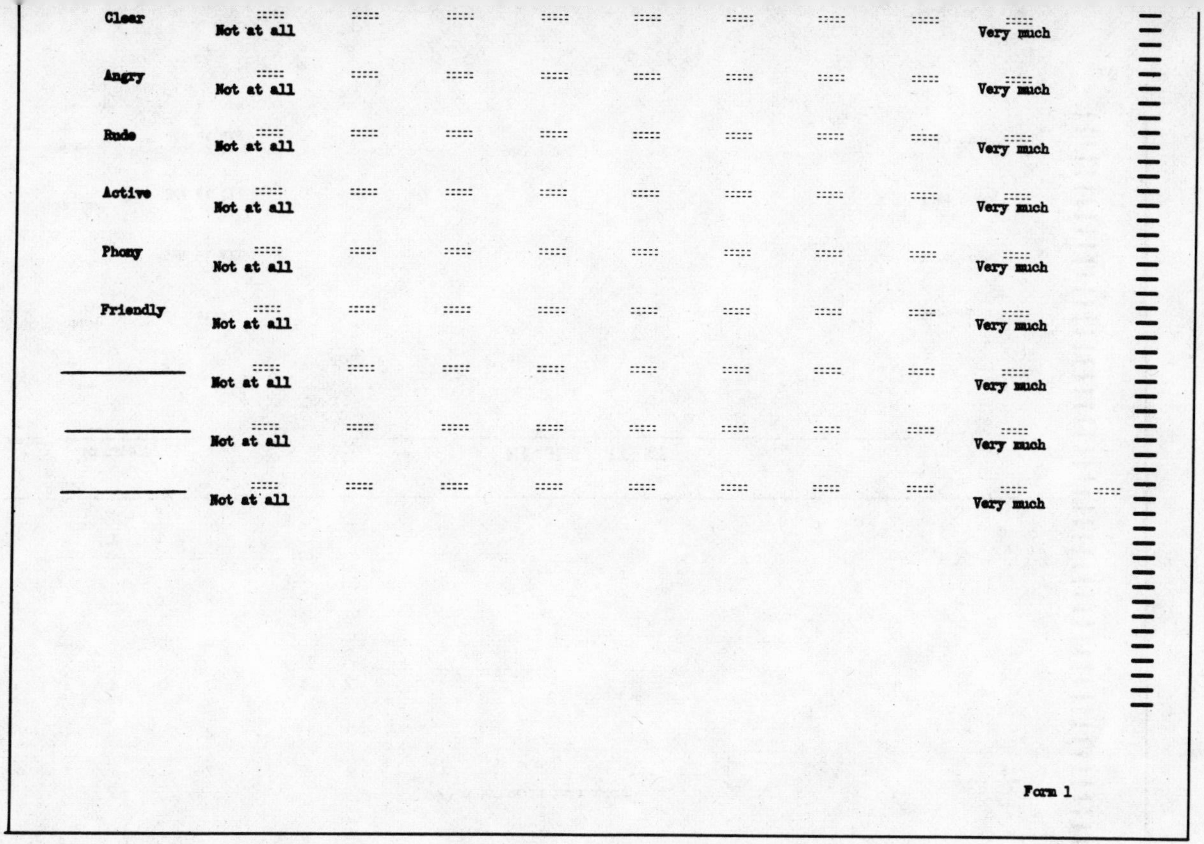

Clear   Not at all .... Very much
Angry   Not at all .... Very much
Rude   Not at all .... Very much
Active   Not at all .... Very much
Phony   Not at all .... Very much
Friendly Not at all .... Very much
_____ Not at all .... Very much
_____ Not at all .... Very much
_____ Not at all .... Very much

Form 1

Figure 2. Sample sheet: Family Adjective Rating Scale.

41

Date _____

Do not write in this space

0 1 2 3 4 5 6 7 8 9

F N Qm Qt

A F S H

C T L N

Rater **(Mother)**

MY SON, JIMMY

Active	Not at all	Very much
Bored	Not at all	Very much
Patient	Not at all	Very much
Rude	Not at all	Very much

42

Afraid	Not at all	:::::	:::::	:::::	:::::	:::::	:::::	:::::	:::::	:::::	Very much
Controlling	Not at all	:::::	:::::	:::::	:::::	:::::	:::::	:::::	:::::	:::::	Very much
Phony	Not at all	:::::	:::::	:::::	:::::	:::::	:::::	:::::	:::::	:::::	Very much
Friendly	Not at all	:::::	:::::	:::::	:::::	:::::	:::::	:::::	:::::	:::::	Very much
Angry	Not at all	:::::	:::::	:::::	:::::	:::::	:::::	:::::	:::::	:::::	Very much
Clear	Not at all	:::::	:::::	:::::	:::::	:::::	:::::	:::::	:::::	:::::	Very much
____________	Not at all	:::::	:::::	:::::	:::::	:::::	:::::	:::::	:::::	:::::	Very much
____________	Not at all	:::::	:::::	:::::	:::::	:::::	:::::	:::::	:::::	:::::	Very much
____________	Not at all	:::::	:::::	:::::	:::::	:::::	:::::	:::::	:::::	:::::	Very much

Form 2

Figure 2. (Continued)

read aloud by the project worker. This individual oral administration always was used with children.

One of six random orders of adjectives was presented for each concept and the six concepts were rated in standard order, as discussed in Appendix A, p. 237. Some differences in procedures in the two data collection years are also described there.

Factor analyses of the adjective ratings indicate that all raters adopted globally positive and negative orientations in making their judgments. Repeated factor analyses using different pilot groups yielded two factors which emerged consistently. The first was an interpersonal activity factor with strongly negative evaluations. This included high positive loadings for the three adjectives *angry, phony,* and *rude* and a high negative loading for *patient.* These negative characteristics seem to imply strong impact on others; that is, the potency connotations are also high.

The second factor represented the obverse: highly positive characteristics of active interpersonal behavior, including high positive loadings on *friendly, active,* and *controlling,* and a negative loading on *bored.* Again the implication of strong effect on others is suggested, this time of a positive character. It is of interest that both factors include only manifest activity or outwardly directed aspects of behavior. Neither "afraid," implying shrinking, inhibited behavior, nor "clear," connoting the quality of communication, had consistent loadings in factor analyses.

Since all adjectives were used to rate persons, the factors are seen as referring to the individual's perceived social impact on others. We therefore labeled the first factor as connoting "Negative Social Impact" and the second factor as connoting "Positive Social Impact." Since these factors frequently were replicated (see Appendix A), they are used consistently whenever adjective rating results are reported.

Along the evaluative (positive to negative) dimension, comparisons of group ratings on the two factors permit study of differences in judgments of presumably desirable and undesirable characteristics of impactful interpersonal functioning. Particularly for the interpersonal behavior of schoolchildren, but apparently applying to adults as well, the two factors represent "social effectiveness" and "social symptom" characteristics. These are reasonably independent characteristics, such that a person could be rated the same or different, on both factors, in different interactions or at different times.

The degree to which this evaluative split represents social desirability or other rater sets adopted by the two groups of families is important to consider. Likely degrees of these influences are discussed throughout the report.

The results of adjective ratings made by family members are described in three sets of comparisons derived from analyses of variance: (1) differences between groups (e.g., R/NR); (2) differences associated with family role (fathers, mothers, and children) as raters and "ratees"; and (3) interactions between the two, for example, differences between family members (fathers, mothers, and children) within referred and nonreferred groups as they rate and as they are rated. All ratings were examined separately from two perspectives: once in terms of the ratings made by each person (Table 1), and later in terms of the ratings received by each person (Table 2). The first analyses describe the effects according to the person making the rating: father, mother, or child. Analyses are based on ratings made by 45 R and 27 NR fathers, 59 R and 29 NR mothers, and 60 R and 29 NR children.

Referred—Nonreferred Comparisons

COMPARISONS BASED ON THE PERSON RATING: RATER EFFECTS

Table 1 summarizes six analyses of variance: Group (R/NR) × Person Rated (Fa, Mo, Ch) analyses for each set of raters separately (fathers, mothers, and children); these were computed for each of the two factors (Negative and Positive Social Impact). For each rater, adjective scores were averaged over all the ratings he made (e.g., for fathers: their ratings of themselves, their wives, and their children). (1) The Group (R/NR) effects reflect the differences in ratings made by referred as compared to nonreferred family members (e.g., by R fathers as compared to NR fathers). (2) The Person Rated effect compares the differences in the ratings made of each family member by the three member groups (e.g., for fathers, ratings made by fathers of fathers, mothers, and children, both R and NR). (3) The third entry reflects the differences in the ratings of family members made by referred raters in contrast to the ratings made by their NR counterparts (e , for fathers, differences in R and NR fathers' ratings of family members).

Table 1 shows the direction and degree of statistical significance of the differences obtained through these analyses. The findings are summarized in the text. Results are presented only for differences that are significant at the $p < .10$ level or lower. The statistical data on which these comparisons are based are contained in Appendix B, Table 4.

1. The (R, NR) entry compared referred and nonreferred family members' estimates of themselves and their families. Results show that all three members of referred families gave ratings that were significantly more negative than did the members of control families. The former gave higher ratings on the Negative Social Impact factor and lower ratings on Positive Social Impact. *Such a devaluating use of the adjectives by each member within the referred family suggests a pervasive low level of esteem for the interper-*

Table 1.   Family Adjective Ratings—Rater Effects

	Factor IB: Negative Social Impact		Factor IIB: Positive Social Impact	
Analysis of Variance	a	b	a	b
Father is rater				
Group (R, NR)	NR<R	.001	NR>R	.05
Family member rated (Mo, Fa, Ch)	Mo=Fa<Ch	.001	Mo>Fa>Ch	.01
Group × Member Rated			R: Mo>Fa>Ch NR: Ch>Mo>Fa	.01
Mother is rater				
Group	NR<R	.01	NR>R	.05
Family member rated	Mo<Fa<Ch	.01		
Group × Member Rated			R: Mo>Fa>Ch NR: Ch > Fa > Mo	.05
Child is rater				
Group	NR<R	.01	NR>R	.10
Family member rater	Mo=Fa<Ch	.01	Mo>Fa>Ch	.001
Group × Member Rated			R: Mo>Fa>Ch NR: Fa>Mo>Ch	:10

ᵃ < indicates that the mean for the first mentioned group is smaller than the mean of the second group; > indicates that the first mean is larger than the second.
ᵇ indicates the significance level of the comparisons.

sonal attributes of self and other family members. Whereas the referred parents and children view themselves and their families quite negatively, the control family members reflect relatively "good" feelings about themselves and each other.

It is easily conceivable that the NR families would have a set to report highly positive interpersonal evaluations in this situation. Comparably, referred parents might well share a tendency to devalue the child whose difficulty "brought" them to a psychological clinic, and each might well extend such a negative orientation to include the spouse who is then seen as failing to perform adequately in his or her parental function. In the same way, self-devaluing, guilty reactions often appear in verbalizations of parents when their children have been identified as disturbed. Even while allowing for such possible set effects, however, the highly uniform character and direction of *all* group ratings reported here would still seem noteworthy.

2. The second component of rater effects (the Person Rated, combining referred and nonreferred family members), contrasted the ratings each rater group gave to all family members. In this way evaluations made of each person by fathers, by mothers, and by children were examined separately. Two overall differences emerged in these comparisons in Table 1.

(a) *All three groups of raters indicated that children were seen more negatively than adults.* They were rated as behaving "badly" (high on Negative Social Impact) and ineffectively (low on Positive Social Impact). This finding probably reflects the children's status in the family and the fact that they have not completed the social learning process as it is prescribed by adults. As raters, children indicated their awareness of their deficiencies in this regard and expressed their lower self-perceptions in comparison to their parents' self-ratings.

(b) *Fathers and children concurred in the evaluative judgments they expressed for both parents, whereas mothers rated differently.* Fathers and children described the two parents as equal in their rude, phony, or impatient behaviors but mothers termed themselves as "better" than their husbands in this regard; that is, they gave themselves lower negativity ratings. Fathers and children also agreed in appraising the mother as the most effective social agent in the family (highest Positive Impact) but the mothers again diverged, rating themselves not significantly higher than they rated their husbands on this score. (Whereas fathers and children gave the sequence Mo > Fa > Ch, the mothers' rating pattern was Mo = Fa > Ch.) Whether the mothers were being modest, genuinely felt less adequate, or saw themselves as more passive, thus matching their self-concept of "goodness," (low self-ratings on negativity) is not known. In any case, mothers clearly rated themselves differently from the congruent views held of them by fathers and children. Since there were four times as many boys as girls in this child sample, this father-child agreement may be largely due to sex identification.

3. Analysis for each rater of the interaction between his group (R or NR) and the person he was rating (father, mother, child) reflects the extent to which referred and nonreferred family members differed in the scores they assigned to themselves and other family members. It appears from Table 1 that such differences were greater in the attribution of positive than negative interpersonal characteristics. For the negative factor there were no significant interactions in the ratings made by fathers, mothers, or children. For Positive Social Impact, however, there were significant Group × Person Rated interactions in all three sets of ratings. Thus *the relative amount of Positive Social Impact assigned to family members was significantly different for referred as compared to nonreferred father, mother, and child*

groups. Each of the three referred raters produced an identical pattern in which the highest valuation for social effectiveness was assigned to mother, second to father, and lowest to child (by fathers at $p < .01$, by mothers at $p < .05$, and by children at $p < .10$). *In nonreferred families, on the other hand, both parents viewed the child as highest in interpersonal competence and each gave second place to the spouse.*

Since the referred children were present because their behavior previously had been judged inadequate, it was to be expected that they would be seen unfavorably. And since the nonreferred children had been identified as having no major social problems, it is possible that their parents' high evaluations of them reflected this influence, perhaps even on a temporary or situational basis. However, *the concurrence of all referred family members in rating the mother as more socially effective than the father may reflect genuine differences in perception of relative parental competence or social power.* By contrast, the nonreferred parents each seemed to defer to the other by consistently rating themselves least favorably, perhaps because they perceived greater adequacy in the other. A possible inference, that the mutually highly valuation expressed between control parents implies higher levels of mutual respect and confidence than was reflected in the families of referred children, receives additional support from other measures.

It is interesting that there are greater differences between the two sets of families in their expression of positive attributions than in their mutual disparagements. *Interpersonal difficulty of the kind being studied here seems more than a manifestation of negative feeling; it also reflects a lower level of mutual friendly involvement, activity, and interpersonal responsiveness.*

COMPARISONS BASED ON THE PERSON BEING RATED: PERSON RATED EFFECTS

The *ratings received by* each family member were compared for R versus NR groups; the ratings made of each family member by each rater group were compared for all families, R + NR; and again the interactions of Group (R, NR) × Person Rating for the ratings received by each family member were studied. Table 2 shows the direction of all group differences that reach at least $p < .10$ level of significance. (See Appendix B, Table 5 for statistical data).

1. The (R, NR) group effect shows the extent to which referred and nonreferred families differed in the ratings received by each member. These analyses combine the fathers', mothers', and children's ratings of individual members (e.g., of the father). The table shows that the ratings given to all three nonreferred family members were less negative on the Negative Social Impact factor than ratings given the referred family members ($p < .001$).

Table 2. Family Adjective Ratings—Person Rated Effects

Analysis of Variance	Factor IB: Negative Social Impact		Factor IIB: Positive Social Impact	
	a	*b*	*a*	*b*
Ratings of fathers				
Group	NR<R	.001	NR>R	.001
Rater (Mo, Fa, Ch)	Ch<Mo=Fa	.05		
Group × Rater			R: Ch>Fa>Mo	.05
			NR: Ch=Mo>Fa	
Ratings of mother				
Group	NR<R	.001		
Rater	Ch<Mo=Fa	.10		
Group × Rater				
Ratings of child				
Group	NR<R	.002	NR>R	.001
Rater	Ch<Mo=Fa	.01		
Group × Rater				

a < indicates that the mean for the first mentioned group is smaller than the mean of the second group; > indicates that the first mean is larger than the second.
b indicates the significance level of the comparisons.

Also, on the Positive Social Impact factor, nonreferred fathers and children received higher ratings than their referred counterparts ($p < .001$). Thus, just as all raters in referred families had expressed lower esteem for themselves and their families in the ratings they made, the combined "ratings received" analysis showed that *all three referred family members were described in relatively negative* (high Negative Impact) *and inadequate* (low Positive Impact) *terms. The one exception was that referred mothers were rated by themselves and their families at the same level of Positive Social Impact as the nonreferred mothers.* A smiling, encouraging motherhood stereotype could be involved here; or there could be, in fact, no difference between mother groups; or referred mothers may be "bad" (rude, angry, phony, and impatient) and yet still operate with high social effectiveness. Additional data from other measures in this study will help to clarify this question.

The child was seen as being more like the father than like the mother in ratings by all family members. Again, sex identification on the part of the 81% boys in the referred sample may have produced this result.

2. The way in which family groups (father, mother, and child) ordered the different members is indicated by the "rater" components of the per-

son rated effect. This provided an assessment of relative family position or status as seen by the person making the rating (independent of the referred, nonreferred classification). There were no role differences evidenced for the positive factor but children rated everyone less severely on negativity than did the parents. Mothers and fathers tended to be quite similar in their descriptions of negative attributes of all the family.

The simplest interpretation of this finding is that adults were in agreement about the relatively high levels of socialization they had achieved in comparison with their children. Particularly, they described themselves as exercising greater control over expression of negative affect and saw the children as still far from exhibiting conformity to cultural expectations in this regard. The children's ratings may have reflected either their relative noninvolvement in negative evaluative processes, or perhaps a quite understandable leaning toward tolerance and charity on this score.

3. The interaction of Group (R, NR) × Rater (Fa, Mo, Ch) in this "family member being rated" analysis indicates the extent to which individual raters in the two groups differed in appraising each member of the family. Only one statistically significant interaction was found. On the Positive Social Impact factor, referred family members rated the father differently than did nonreferred family members. *Children in both groups gave the highest positive ratings to the father.* In nonreferred families, the mother gave a similarly high rating to her husband, who gave himself the most modest rating of the three. In referred families, fathers rated themselves higher than their wives did, the latter providing the lowest evaluation of the three ratings given the father. *Thus in referred families, fathers tend to be devalued by their wives relative to their own self-ratings, whereas in nonreferred families wives tend to express higher valuation for the father than he attributes to himself.* Again, as in the "rater effect" analysis (Table 1), the expressed appraisal of the father's positive attributes differentiates between referred and nonreferred families. There is a lower expression of confidence in their husbands' social strengths on the part of referred mothers, in contrast to controls.

It is evident that on this measure, contrasts between fathers in the referred and nonreferred families were greater than the differences between the referred and control children, who constituted the basis for classification into the two groups. The salience of the role of the father in the two groups seems manifest, especially in the differential view of the father's status in the family vis-à-vis his wife.

An overview of ratings *made by* and ratings *received by* all family members (Tables 1 and 2) shows that in 11 out of the 12 basic R/NR comparisons, the referred member was always significantly lower on expressed social valuation than the nonreferred counterpart. There were no reversals. In the twelfth comparison, there was no significant difference in ratings of mothers' Positive Impact between the two groups. Possible implication for perceived maternal social superiority in referred families has been mentioned.

To the extent that their use of these adjectives does in fact reflect peoples' perceptions of themselves and each other, results suggest that there are very significant and generalized differences in the favorableness of personal and interpersonal regard expressed within the two sets of families. To the extent to which the ratings reflect only relatively negative or positive response sets within the two groups of families, results suggest that the quality of input each family member receives from others is significantly more positive in control families and more negative in referreds. The consistency of the results is especially notable since other studies of parents' perceptions of each other often have failed to find a difference between families of disturbed and normal control children (e.g., Frank, 1965; Becker, 1959).

EXPECTATIONS OF HOW OTHERS WILL RATE

In separate ratings each member of the family triad estimated how he would be perceived by the other two. Table 3 presents the means and the p level of t tests between referred and nonreferred groups.

The entries in this table show that in all comparisons, *members of referred families expected higher negativity and lower effectiveness ratings from both other family members than did the members of control families.* The differences between groups were statistically significant in nine of the 12 comparisons. The three that did not achieve statistical significance followed patterns that had been observed in other relationships: (1) though

Table 3. Family Adjective Ratings—Mean Expectations of How Members of the Family Will Rate Each Other

	Factor IB: Negative Social Impact			Factor IIB: Positive Social Impact		
	R	NR	$p<$	R	NR	$p<$
Fa rating						
How child will rate	4.42	3.39	.01	5.32	6.04	.01
How wife will rate	4.24	3.39	.01	5.07	5.46	ns
Mo rating						
How child will rate	4.61	3.71	.01	4.87	5.76	.01
How husband will rate	4.31	3.82	ns	4.75	5.03	ns
Ch rating						
How father will rate	3.92	3.11	.05	4.74	5.47	.05
How mother will rate	4.22	3.19	.01	4.50	5.57	.001

referred fathers expected their wives to rate them significantly high on rudeness, anger, etc., they anticipated positive ratings of their interpersonal effectiveness. This optimistic anticipation turned out to be inaccurate, for their wives rated them relatively negatively on both factors. (2) and (3) In contrast, the referred mother evidently felt secure in her expectations of her husband's favorable ratings of her, as her anticipations were comparable to those of the nonreferred mothers on both factors (the group means were not significantly different). These three nonsignificant findings, taken together, support the earlier suggestion that *referred mothers can and do expect to be more highly rated by their husbands than the latter can in turn expect from their wives.* Again, the referred wife has the advantage in status over her husband.

In summary, the anticipation of relatively poor ratings expressed by each member of the families of referred children was realized amply, just as the more sanguine estimates of control families were borne out. In general, mutual evaluations were predicted with remarkable accuracy.

In all findings, adjective ratings by family members explicated very consistently and significantly the differences in positive and negative expression of interpersonal evaluation that distinguished families of children who had adapted well at school from families of children whose behavior was manifestly troubled. *The quality of the child's interpersonal adaptation in the school setting seems related to the appraisals of interpersonal adequacy and respect expressed within the family.*

To the extent that reported differences are based on rater sets, these would appear to be learned by children at early ages and maintained in a wide variety of conditions (e.g., in specifying expectations as to how others will rate). Some of the consistent findings such as the higher Positive Impact uniformly assigned to mothers in referred families and to fathers in nonreferred families are hard to interpret entirely within a rater set framework.

Socioeconomic Level Comparisons of Family Adjective Rating Scales

COMPARISONS BASED ON THE PERSON RATING: RATER EFFEECTS

SEL membership did not markedly influence family members' use of the adjective scales. In Rater $\times$ Socioeconomic Level analyses of variance, there were no significant main effects.

One significant ($p < .05$) SEL $\times$ Person Rated interaction appeared for the Negative Social Impact factor. This occurred in ratings made by mothers. Hi and Mid SEL mothers rated themselves and their husbands less negatively than they rated their children; Lo SEL mothers' ratings were in the order self < child < husband. This is consistent with the earlier analysis which indicated that all parents rate themselves less negatively than they rate their children. When it is recalled that more than half of the Lo SEL mothers had no husbands, it is reasonable that these mothers should rate themselves as least negative (from the usual adult perspective), with the child in second place since the absent husband would doubtless be viewed in highly negative terms. In the absence of a main effect, this single interaction is noted only since it fits into the obvious consequences of the single-parent condition.

Analysis of variance for (R, NR) × SEL ratings for each rater on each factor yielded no significant interactions. *We thus conclude that families at all SEL levels experience and express their interpersonal regard in a similar fashion, at least in terms of their use of adjective scales.* Apparently economic and sociocultural factors did not determine the favorable versus unfavorable expression of interpersonal evaluation within families. Methodologically this finding suggests that the use of definitions and explanatory techniques used in the administration of the adjective scales had resulted in a task that was meaningful for parents and children at all educational levels represented in our sample.

COMPARISONS BASED ON THE PERSON BEING RATED:
PERSON RATED EFFECTS

Hi SEL fathers received higher ratings for their Positive Social Impact than did Lo SEL fathers ($p < .05$). There was a trend ($p < .10$) for Mid SEL children to be rated lowest of the three child groups on social effectiveness. These two isolated findings are reported here since they receive statistical support and a meaningful context in the results of other measures. No significant rater effects or Rater × SEL interactions were obtained.

Referral Category Comparisons

When adjective ratings of referred children were classified into groups on the basis of each child's predominant problem, there were no statistically significant referral category effects in any analysis of variance. *No pattern of Positive or Negative Social Impact, as reflected in adjective ratings, was associated with any type of behavioral difficulty shown by the referred children. Their development of the specific patterns of interpersonal symptomatology displayed in the school setting appears to be triggered and maintained on bases other than the generalized unfavorable regard expressed within the referred families.*

PARENT BEHAVIOR INVENTORY

Items in this questionnaire sampled mothers' and fathers' separate ratings of (1) their child's behavior and their own actions in relation to him, (2) their activities and relationship with each other, and (3) their involvement and satisfaction with their community. Questions were intended to ascertain where, when, and how often observable behaviors occurred. No attempt was made to get historical data: parental memories with respect to children's developmental data seem generally unreliable (e.g., Robbins, 1963; Hoffman, 1960) and our interest was in current perceptions and behavior. No questions tapped generalized attitudes since inquiries about concrete behavioral events appear to yield more reliable data than reports of attitudes and feelings (Haggard et al., 1961; Fontana, 1966). Also, it was assumed that attitudinal factors would be major components of the adjective ratings which parents made separately. Questionnaire items were couched in terms that were as concrete as possible in an attempt to reduce ambiguity of the scales and to set up specific reference points for time, place, and frequency of interpersonal situations.

The standard procedure was for each parent to be given a copy of the Behavior Inventory at the conclusion of the first interview. Mothers and fathers were requested to fill out their questionnaires separately and bring them in at their second appointment. The forms consisted of 101 items covering 33 pages; the topics were arranged in different sequences in fathers' and mothers' forms, making parental collaboration exceedingly difficult. Whenever there was any question of a parent's ability to comprehend the items, an additional appointment was scheduled and the inventory was filled out at the clinic with the assistance of a project worker. Despite these efforts, some inventories were not returned, or were incomplete. Reported analyses are based on inventories of 28 R, 25 NR fathers and 41 R, 26 NR mothers.

The format of the Inventory is illustrated in Figure 3, which reproduces a sample page of questions about the child's specific behaviors. All the items in the Inventory and the results of the factor analytic methods used to cluster the items in the inventory are contained in Appendix A, pp. 242-244.

One part of the inventory sampled the *child's behavior in the context of the family*. Included in this part were questions about his activity, self-sufficiency, and instrumental effectiveness (task orientation, responsible work performance, autonomous behavior); his interpersonal adaptiveness (activity level, responsiveness to parents, affectionate behavior, sociability); his ways of expressing aggression and hostility; and his tendencies to withdraw from social interactions (e.g., fearfulness, crying, solitary play). Another part covered topics emphasizing *parental behavior in relation to the child*. These included amounts of affectionate behavior; amounts of interaction, communication, closeness, and understanding; ways in which the parent seeks to influence and discipline the child; and ways in which the parent expresses anger toward the child. A third category of topics focused on the *parents in relationship to each other and to their local community*, through questions about how decisions were made in the family, how the parents sought to influence each other, and how they resolved disagreements. Family role behavior was explored by examining the extent to which different family members engaged in various household activities. The relation of family members to the community was assessed by inquiring into their participation in formal and informal community groups.

These topics seemed to encompass most of the behaviors generally considered important in the child development and family process literature. In this discussion they are considered in the light of their relationship to the basic interpersonal dimensions studied throughout the project: (1) interpersonal evaluation (positive or negative); (2) high or low activity levels and direct or indirect activity styles; and (3) the range and characteristics of attempts at interpersonal influence. Assessment of the effect of interpersonal influence is necessarily inferential in this as in our other measures. Since the items of the inventory are descriptions of behaviors, not interactions, the discussions of effects of influence efforts are restricted to other responses which indicate how family members responded to the interpersonal influence techniques reported. For example, a father's report that his child repeatedly ignores his scolding would imply that the father's verbal efforts at control are ineffective.

As with the other instruments, Parent Behavior Inventories were compared for parental responses (*a*) in referred as compared to control families, (*b*) in families grouped acording to SEL, and (*c*) in families grouped in terms of the child's predominant type of behavioral problem (Referral Category). Analyses were computed by assigning factor scores to individual responses. Mothers' and fathers' responses were factored separately (Kaiser Varimax rotation; see Appendix A) because the resulting factors accounted for more of the total variance than when mothers' and fathers' responses were combined. In general, the meaning of items in mother and father factors were very similar although there rarely was complete overlap in the item composition of factors (see Appendix A).

As mentioned, the inventory was factored in three different sections. One contained the items describing *relations of the parents to each other and the family's relation to the community*. Analysis of this section yielded 9 factors for father's and 10 factors for mother's inventories. Another set of items described the *parent's behavior in relation to the child*. This yielded 10 factors for the mother's and 8 for the father's inventories. The third set contained the *parent's report of the child's behavior toward him*. Both mother's and father's inventories yielded 15 factors for this section.

These three sections are presented in the text under sequential headings: Parent → Spouse, Parent → Child, and Child → Parent Behaviors. Under each heading, descriptions and/or illustrative items are listed for all factors

15. How often does your child do the following:

(a) Cry

At most several times a year	About once a month	About once a week	Almost every day	Several times a day

(b) Whine and complain

At most several times a year	About once a month	About once a week	Almost every day	Several times a day

(c) Get angry

At most several times a year	About once a month	About once a week	Almost every day	Several times a day

(d) Get fidgety

At most several times a year	About once a month	About once a week	Almost every day	Several times a day

(e) Go off by himself

At most several times a year	About once a month	About once a week	Almost every day	Several times a day

(f) Get extra quiet

At most several times a year	About once a month	About once a week	Almost every day	Several times a day

56

(g) Get silly	At most several times a year	About once a month	About once a week	Almost every day	Several times a day
(h) Do his work poorly	At most several times a year	About once a month	About once a week	Almost every day	Several times a day
(i) Go to mother for comfort	At most several times a year	About once a month	About once a week	Almost every day	Several times a day
(j) Go to father for comfort	At most several times a year	About once a month	About once a week	Almost every day	Several times a day
(k) Have temper tantrums	At most several times a year	About once a month	About once a week	Almost every day	Several times a day
(l) Complain that something hurts him	At most several times a year	About once a month	About once a week	Almost every day	Several times a day

Figure 3. Sample sheet: Parent Behavior Inventory.

Child Study Program
Psychology - UCLA

78. How often does each member of the family do gardening or yard work?

(a) Husband

::::: At most several times a year | ::::: About once a month | ::::: About once a week | ::::: Almost every day | ::::: Several times a day

(b) Wife

::::: At most several times a year | ::::: About once a month | ::::: About once a week | ::::: Almost every day | ::::: Several times a day

(c) Child

::::: At most several times a year | ::::: About once a month | ::::: About once a week | ::::: Almost every day | ::::: Several times a day

79. How often does each of you fix things around the house?

(a) Husband

::::: At most several times a year | ::::: About once a month | ::::: About once a week | ::::: Almost every day | ::::: Several times a day

(b) Wife

::::: At most several times a year | ::::: About once a month | ::::: About once a week | ::::: Almost every day | ::::: Several times a day

(c) Child

At most several times a year | About once a month | About once a week | Almost every day | Several times a day

80. How often does each of you carry out trash and do clean-up jobs?

(a) Husband

At most several times a year | About once a month | About once a week | Almost every day | Several times a day

(b) Wife

At most several times a year | About once a month | About once a week | Almost every day | Several times a day

(c) Child

At most several times a year | About once a month | About once a week | Almost every day | Several times a day

81. How often do you and your husband do the following:

(a) Discuss the children

At most several times a year | About once a month | About once a week | Almost every day | Several times a day

Figure 3. (Continued)

59

that resulted in significant differentiation or trends ($p < .10$) between groups. Groups of factors that are conceptually related (e.g., Interpersonal Closeness) are labeled to help organize the data. All the factors and the results of the various comparisons are summarized in Table 4.

Referred—Nonreferred Comparisons

PARENT-SPOUSE BEHAVIOR

Father→Mother (father's responses specifying the frequency of his behaviors and activities with his wife)

Share decisions and activities	NR > R	$p < .01$
Hostile disagreements and wide range of interpersonal influence attempts (both direct and indirect, "forceful" and "tentative")	R > NR	$p < .01$

Father→Community

Likes neighborhood and neighbors	NR > R	$p < .05$

Mother→Father (mother's responses specifying the frequency of her behaviors with her husband)

Share decisions and activities	NR > R	$p < .01$
One parent decides alone	R > NR	$p < .01$
Hostile disagreement; forceful attempts at interpersonal influence	R > NR	$p < .05$

Mother→Community

Likes neighborhood and neighbors	NR > R	$p < .05$

The nonreferred mothers and fathers agree in reporting many shared decision and activity patterns. The generally positive feeling expressed between the parents extends to their community, from which they gain satisfaction, and to their neighbors, whom they see as likeable.

The referred parents report disagreement, hostility, and conflict. The fathers describe themselves as frequently using a wide variety of ways in trying to influence their wives. These range from very active, direct power-assertion efforts (for example, "When you want your wife to do something, you get angry if she doesn't do it") to passive, indirect pleas in which they imply feelings of powerlessness ("When you disagree with your wife, you let her know you feel hurt"). Their wives indicate a corresponding involvement in marital dissatisfaction and conflict but emphasize predominantly active, assertive efforts. High frequencies are typical for items like "How often do you and your husband argue?" and "When you want your husband to do something how often do you use the approach that you will be angry if he doesn't do it?". Items suggesting a passive influence stance, like the use of hurt feelings, appear in mothers' responses in a factor which did not differentiate between R and NR mothers. *This stronger demand character of referred wives' responses coupled with the referred fathers' inclusion of more passive influence efforts suggests that the referred mothers may have higher status positions within the family than do their husbands.* This repeats the pattern of relatively high Positive Social Impact assigned to referred mothers (over fathers) in the Family Adjective Ratings.

For both referred parents, the dissatisfaction with the marital relationship is accompanied by a dislike of neighbors and the local community. The overall picture is of people experiencing dissatisfaction and discontent with their general life situation. These responses thus confirm the adjective ratings, where they had also expressed lower evaluations of themselves and each other than had nonreferred parents.

For mothers' responses, the significant factor indicating that one parent makes decisions alone undoubtedly is weighted heavily by the single-parent families and is discussed in that context, in SEL comparisons.

FATHER-CHILD BEHAVIOR

Father→Child (father's responses describing the child and his own behavior with him)

Interpersonal closeness and activity		
Father shares activities with child, works, plays, and jokes with him	NR > R	$p < .01$
Father understands child's thoughts and feelings, sees him as like wife	NR > R	$p < .01$
Father reports that child talks, works, and plays with him	NR > R	$p < .05$
Discipline and influence attempts		
Father ignores, physically isolates child as punishment	R > NR	$p < .06$
Father uses personalized, referent influence attempts: asks child to perform for father's sake	R > NR	$p < .06$
Father gets angry, yells, hits, scolds, shames	R > NR	$p < .01$

Child→Father (father's responses describing child and child's behavior towards him)

Child is seen as task oriented and independent	NR > R	$p < .05$
Child is seen as highly responsive to paternal attention, approval, and disapproval	NR > R	$p < .05$
Child is seen as athletic, noisy, talkative	NR > R	$p < .05$
Child cries, whines, blames others, lacks autonomy	R > NR	$p < .05$
Child avoids personal confrontations, is tense, fearful, hostile, manipulative	R > NR	$p < .05$
Child is sensitive to interpersonal ridicule and unfairness; has somatic complaints	R > NR	$p < .01$
Child is hostile and defiant to father, verbally and physically	R > NR	$p < .01$
Child is verbally hostile to peers, threatens, and quarrels	R > NR	$p < .01$

The nonreferred father's relations with his child are characterized by a high degree of interpersonal activity and psychological closeness: the nonreferred father is actively involved with the child, enjoys being with him, sees him as like the mother and reports him to have highly desirable attributes of independence, self-reliance, and task orientation. He does not raise significant complaints or seem anxious about him. The father does not report any special form of discipline but the effectiveness of his paternal role and power is manifested in the child's responsiveness to paternal approval and disapproval. The relationship and the child are reported in positive, directly active terms, with little concern about discipline or interpersonal influence.

The referred father's relations with his child are characterized by largely negative values in his descriptions of the child's behavior. These fathers are much concerned about their attempt to discipline, influence, and control the child. They have little actual contact with the child, do not feel close to him, and don't seem to enjoy him. In their disciplinary efforts they report using three quite different methods: *(a)* punishment through exclusion and inattention (the direct opposite of the positive, shared activity described by control fathers); *(b)* rationalized attempts to use the affectional relationship to get the child to behave in a desired way (through implication of guilt, responsibility, etc.); and *(c)* angry outbursts, including shouting and hitting.

A pervasive negative evaluation colors the referred father's attempts at influencing the child. Activity and potency levels appear to vary together in two patterns. The first manifests a low or indirect type of activity, along with the assumption of a low power position. It is characterized by the father's rationalized, complaining, conciliatory efforts to get the child to be active and responsible (to meet the parent's need to have him behave in a certain way). The second pattern involves explosive anger, the father being highly active and very demanding of the child. Analyses thus far do not indicate whether these results represent different subgroups within the total referred fathers; alternatively, some fathers may use one or the other pattern exclusively for a period of time or may fluctuate between the two. In any case, within the total referred group, the father reports trying everything: he ignores, rationalizes, attempts to elicit sympathy or induce guilt, conciliates, pleads, scolds, yells, and hits. Fluctuations across such a range of behaviors imply that none is producing the desired effect. And this is in fact what referred fathers describe: the child does not behave as the father wants him to; the father cannot control and influence the child as much as either he wants to or feels he should. In his efforts to demonstrate parental power while feeling psychologically distant from the child, he has been ineffective.

As the referred father itemizes his complaints about his offspring's behavior, it becomes clear that *the child employs many of the behavioral styles his father has manifested.* (This is at least the picture conveyed in paternal reports of child behavior). The father's low activity and low power position are mirrored in the child when he cries, whines, blames others, avoids confrontation, is sensitive, and is nonautonomous. The father's angry explosions have their counterpart in the child's talking back, in his verbal and physical attacks on the parent. Although our data do not depict specific interactional patterns, we speculate that the two stances may sometimes be adopted by parent and child in see-saw fashion: when one is high, the other is low. In other situations they may become intermingled, building in long continuous spirals or occurring in brief episodic cycles. Whatever the interactional pattern, both father and child clearly manifest a similar wide range of interpersonal influence attempts, and the basic issue of who is in control remains unresolved. A vivid picture of the child's modeling of the father seems contained in these data; counterreactions reflecting the adoption of opposing behavior styles may also be involved. Data from behavioral samples in the next chapter depict further differentiations in these father-child patterns.

MOTHER-CHILD BEHAVIOR

Mother→Child (mother's responses describing the child and her own behavior with him)

Legitimate, referent, personalized influence techniques (it's the child's duty to obey; the mother will be hurt, etc.)   R > NR $p < .05$

Rationalized discipline: make sure child knows what's wrong before you punish; explain, wait till you are not angry   R > NR $p < .05$

Anger: yell, hit, scold   R > NR $p < .01$

Child→Mother (mother's responses describing child and child's response toward her)

Child is seen as task oriented: persists and does well	NR > R	$p < .01$
Child is seen as reactive to maternal affection, praise, rewards	NR > R	$p < .05$
Child is seen as interpersonally active, making friends, not being alone	NR > R	$p < .05$
Child is seen as manipulative, making his performance contingent on rewards	R > NR	$p < .01$
Child is seen as fearful; bites nails	R > NR	$p < .01$
Child is seen as avoiding people, being tense, having somatic reactions	R > NR	$p < .01$
Child is seen as being defiant, talking back to parents, raising complaints	R > NR	$p < .01$
Child is seen as overtly hostile to peers, hitting and hurting others	R > NR	$p < .01$

In responses concerning general activity and closeness with their children, there is no difference between nonreferred and referred mothers. This is in marked contrast to the control fathers' description of the active behavioral involvement which differentiates them from referred fathers. In their descriptions of their child and his behavior toward themselves, however, nonreferred mothers differ from referreds on the same number of factors their husbands had identified. The significant behaviors were, in fact, almost identical in mother and father versions. *The control mothers describe their children as task oriented; as responsive to their efforts to reward or punish them; and as interpersonally active, independent, and friendly.* Though these nonreferred mothers reported less activity with their children than had their husbands, the mother-child dyads still seem to influence and please each other through their manifestation of mutual regard. Parental status is a *fait accompli*; control is not in question.

Referred mothers, in contrast, describe activities associated with disciplinary and control efforts that range from verbal appeals and rational explanations to physical expressions of anger. In their descriptions of their children's behavior toward them, referred mothers depict fearful, tense, defiant, hostile, and hurtful children. And they have a special complaint, not expressed by their husbands, that their children are manipulative and will perform only on a contingency basis.

In this inventory, as in the FARS, both referred parents expressed highly negative evaluations of their children. However, the referred mothers were similar to the nonreferred mothers in stating that they understood their children and shared many activities with them. This is in contrast to the referred fathers who often seemed uncertain, inept, and very much out of touch with their children.

The behavior which contrasts referred and nonreferred children is reported by their parents in ways consistent with all foregoing descriptions. Nonreferred parents emphasize their children's desirable behaviors, while referred parents report complaints, anxieties, and objections. These are specified in terms that validate the school's identification of the child's problems, indicating that the parents see difficulties comparable to the referral categories: *the children are not task oriented* (they do not persist at or complete tasks: Attention Control); *they show symptoms of Social Withdrawal* (they are fearful, tense, avoidant of interpersonal contact); *they are aggressive verbally and physically hostile* (Aggression); *they are nervous, fidgety, and don't get along well with other children* (Hyperactivity).

For control children's behavior, both nonreferred parents place special value on the child's independent task orientation, his willingness and ability to work effectively and well on his own. Within the control families, mothers note the fact that their children have friends, indicating concern with social values, whereas their husbands are more involved in the child's physical activities, in athletic, noisy, talkative behavior, with higher peer-power implications.

The complaining descriptions of both referred parents concur in their rejection of the child's overt hostile behavior. Both report the child's angry defiance to parents and his hurtful behavior to peers, siblings, and others. Such negatively toned, highly active, and manipulative behaviors are strongly condemned by both parents, though they themselves have explicitly exemplified them. By the same token, these parents complain about an alternative extreme, which they also have demonstrated for their children, of assuming low activity, low power positions. The mother notes that the child is fearful, that he is tense and sullen, while the father reports that the child cries, blames others, avoids confrontation, and is sensitive to critcism. The parents' responses imply that they have either the obligation, need, or right to criticize, exclude, punish, or otherwise control the child to extents they have not yet attained.

It should be emphasized that these statements relate only to the specific patterns of factors that differentiated the referred and nonreferred parents in our inventory responses. The complete inventory (Appendix B) covers many expressions of love and concern within families. *There were no differences between R/NR groups in responding to the items that made up fac-*

tors describing warmth, love, and the exchange of affectionate behavior be-tween parents and children. The general impression gained is that referred parents love but do not admire or enjoy their children. This applies particularly to the fathers since as noted, there was no significant difference between referred and nonreferred mothers in sharing a wide range of activities with the child and feeling that they understood him well. Indeed, the possibility arises that the relatively negative, conflictual relationship the referred mothers describe with their husbands may have led them to seek compensatory closeness with the child.

It should also be noted that the referred children seemed to be given as much autonomy as the nonreferred children in making their own choices of clothes and friends, indicating that, on the whole, referred youngsters were not especially infantilized or protected from self-guided experiences. We speculate that these parents, especially the fathers, appear to need the child to be strong in outside relationships. At the same time they want the child's dependence and compliance in relation to themselves as a means of bolstering their own sense of parental effectiveness and power. As these contradictory requirements cannot be met, the father becomes increasingly querulous, contributing to a family atmosphere of anxious irritability. Anecdotally it often seemed that these fathers were somehow under a special pressure to prove something or to live up to something in their own and their wives' expectations that they could never quite attain. This notion is supported by the pattern of adjective ratings between referred spouses and by data reported in the next chapter.

In terms of the child's development, the question of the personal and interpersonal adequacy of the father would seem to have special significance for children in the age range of our sample. It seems probable that in preschool years the child's relationship with his mother may well be paramount, with the quality and consistency of the nurture and structure she provides often representing the central core of his experience. As the child begins to leave the home environment and attempts to cope with the world outside, however, our data suggest that the father exerts critical influence. Additional data on this point are reported in later chapters.

SUMMARY OF R/NR COMPARISONS

Non referred mothers and fathers agree on areas that determine satisfactory parental interaction. These center around the sharing of decisions, activities, and responsibilities, with minimum concern about interpersonal influence or power struggles. The generally positive view expressed within the home tends to extend to the neighborhood. Referred parents report a contrary picture of hostile negative feelings, and a wide range of influence and control struggles that occur in both direct and indirect activity styles. The assumption has long been made that disturbed children are more likely to come from homes where poor marital relations obtain (e.g., Hoffman & Lippett, 1968), and our data substantiate this position. This negativity extends also into dissatisfaction with the neighborhood, resulting in little parental involvement in the community.

The referred child has interpersonal difficulty in his relations with both parents, but the lack of interaction and closeness between the child and his father is striking. It contrasts with the wide range of shared interpersonal activities for control fathers and children, involving knowing, sharing, understanding, working, playing, joking, and talking together. The important criteria relate specifically to what the father reports *doing with* his child, not his attitudes of concern, or his expression of love or warmth.

For many years, the clinical and research literature focused on the mother's influence on child development and behavior. More recently, the importance of the father in affecting children's behavior has begun to be recognized (Peterson et al., 1959; Caputo, 1963). Our results support these later findings, at least for children in this age range, and further indicate some of the specific patterns of father-child relations which differentiate between troubled and socially effective children. But our findings also suggest that a higher maternal status or social power position in the home is associated with the father's failure to fulfill his expected role. This reciprocal interference in role effectiveness, described by Caputo (1963) as role reversal, is discussed further after additional data are introduced.

The R mothers are more active with the children than their husbands are, perhaps, as suggested, in an effort to compensate for their unsatisfactory marital relationship or simply to substitute for the father. The R mothers' activity in this regard exceeds that of the control mothers. The differentiating characteristic of NR mothers is their positive, admiring regard for the child. In the light of the high proportion of boys in this sample, a more passive maternal role could be perceived in the control mothers. This would be in line with a lower level of importance of the mother as a culture-appropriate model for the child's activity at this developmental stage.

Responses of NR parents indicate not only lesser manifestations of undesirable characteristics and behaviors in their children but also the presence of positive attributes such as higher levels of internalized control (the child carries through on his own), and a greater progression toward verbal (symbolic) reinforcements from physical or concrete rewards. There is an implication of generally higher levels of socialization and developmental status for NR as compared to R children. This is in line with Ross's 1963 observation that "good adjustment" is probably something more than the mere absence of maladjustment. It is this lack of perceived personal and social adequacy that is reflected in the relatively low ratings and reports consistently received by R children.

The overall pattern is, quite reasonably, that parents who enjoy satisfactory personal interactions in their marriages have more satisfactory relationships with their children. At least in this sample mothers and fathers who interact to reinforce the fathers' competencies inside and outside the family seem to provide the most suitable models for children at this age. Parents, especially fathers, who reach out, share, and enjoy their contacts with their children have children who feel competent and enjoy working and playing. Parents who exercise clear, consistent influence have responsive, positively reactive children. On the counter side are the parents, especially fathers, who vacillate between demand and entreaty, with both their spouses and children. They have children who show the same wide-ranging, confused, and confusing pattern of interpersonal behavior as their fathers. Such fluctuations seem to reflect a parent's anxious inability to bind his angry, fearful responses and to control himself, his spouse, and most specifically, his child. *This description appears to reflect basically different feelings of personal adequacy and role security in control fathers, relative to the fathers of referred children.*

The results of the Family Adjective Ratings presented earlier indicated that significant evaluative and potency characteristics were differentiated within the two sets of families, with an unknown amount of rater set involved. The same evaluative differentiation was repeated in the Parent Behavior Inventory responses, with negativity predominantly attending referred family interactions, and mutual esteem, respect, and regard reported by control family members. The Behavior Inventory results, however, also delineated in greater detail the different patterns of activity and interpersonal influence styles in the familial transactions of the two groups. These activity and power differences seem harder to explain in terms of raters' sets than the consistent positive-negative evaluative splits reflected on both instruments.

Socioeconomic Level Comparisons

In the R/NR comparisons, despite the relatively low number of father questionnaires (28 referred, 25 nonreferred), the distinguishing role of father-child interactions was evident. Because of the sample distribution of single parents (Chapter 2), SEL comparisons inevitably are weighted heavily by Lo SEL maternal inventories. Fourteen Hi, 31 Mid, and 8 Lo SEL fathers completed Parent Behavior Inventories and 16 Hi, 32 Mid, and 19 Lo SEL mothers completed their forms.

Each factor was analyzed with a SEL × R, NR analysis of variance, but none of the SEL × R, NR interactions reached the .05 p level so that only main effects need be considered. Comparisons involving fathers must be regarded as highly tentative. Since only 4 of the 32 analyses of variance on the father's inventories were significant, the results easily could be due to chance.

PARENT-SPOUSE BEHAVIOR

Father→Mother

Father reports that wife decides alone about money, friends, child — Lo > Mid $p < .05$

Father→Community

Father reports church and home centered activities — Lo > Mid $p < .05$

Mother→Father

Mother describes shared decisions and activities — Hi > Lo $p < .01$ / Mid > Lo $p < .01$

Mother reports disagreement and attempts to influence husband to give in to her — Hi > Mid $p < .05$ / Hi > Lo $p < .05$

Mother reports using personalized influence, nagging, feeling hurt, etc., to get her husband to give in — Hi > Lo $p < .05$

Mother→Community

Mother reports feeling identified with community — Hi > Lo $p < .01$ / Mid > Lo $p < .05$

Lo SEL fathers, when they were physically present in the home, did not exert much influence in familial decision making. Their responses imply a passive, nonassertive role. This finding, of course, may very easily be an artifact of the small N for this father group, but the specific comparisons were congruent with the mothers' responses. There is also considerable likelihood that a highly selective factor involving a generally compliant orientation is represented in this father subsample. Lo SEL fathers typically had little education and evidenced little active interest in clinic services. The willingness of these eight fathers to complete this extensive questionnaire is probably a compliance indicator in itself.

There is a clear Lo SEL single-parent (mother) effect. These women did not report shared parental and marital decisions since over half of them were without husbands. They did not like their community and did in fact tend to live in deteriorating neighborhoods.

Hi SEL mothers made more demands on their husbands than did the other two maternal groups. Whether through disagreement and overt attempts to manipulate, nagging, or appeals to sympathy or sense of obligation, Hi SEL wives tended to assert their own values, position, and needs. This feeling for their individual rights may have been associated with the higher education level generally characteristic of these women.

FATHER-CHILD BEHAVIOR

Father→Child

Father reports use of personalized, referent types of influence; asks child to perform for sake of parent, etc.	Lo > Mid	$p < .05$

Child→Father

Father sees child as autonomous and independent; sees him making his own decisions	Lo > Mid Lo > Hi	$p < .05$ $p < .05$
Father sees child as verbally and physically affectionate	Hi > Lo Hi > Mid	$p < .05$ $p < .05$
Father sees child as responsive to paternal attention, praise, and punishment	Hi > Lo Hi > Mid	$p < .05$ $p < .05$

Differences between Lo and Hi SEL fathers show a distinct contrast in style of influence. The Lo SEL father's method was to approach the child with requests and attempt to motivate him to obey in order to meet his—the father's—needs. The implication is that the child was active, assertive, and independent. The father apparently felt weak relative to both his child and his wife. (This constellation also appears at one end of the wide range of interpersonal influence attempts described by the total group of referred fathers). Again, this finding is not related to feelings of affection and concern expressed by the father for the child. No main SEL effects on this issue appeared either in the adjective ratings or in parent inventory factors designed to tap these areas. However, it would seem likely that the father's ineffectiveness would lead, in time, to a decrease in the family's reliance on and respect for him.

Hi SEL fathers, on the other hand, exceeded both Mid and Lo groups in their reports of receiving affectionate behavior from their children and in feeling that their children were highly responsive to their influence. If these findings are valid, Hi SEL fathers enjoyed a relatively high status and power position with their children. In the preceding section it was noted that Hi SEL mothers felt free to make their needs known to their husbands; these same men received positive feedback and continuing reliance on their judgment from their children. We assume that both maternal freedom to assert prerogatives and the child's warm reactivity would imply and attend paternal ability to meet family needs, conveying to the father a sense of adequacy and competence relative to other fathers. Additional support for this surmise was found in the ratings received by fathers on the Adjective Rating Scales. Hi SEL fathers received higher ratings for their Positive Social Impact than did Lo SEL fathers ($p < .05$). This status is obviously not a uniform attribute of Hi SEL fathers, however, nor does it rule out other sources of interpersonal disturbance in these men. For example, the interpersonal activity items that so clearly distinguished the control fathers were not reported by the Hi SEL fathers as a group. We would assume therefore that Hi SEL condition is neither necessary nor sufficient to ensure the father's effectiveness in his familial roles, but it helps.

These findings with respect to the relationships between the father's power in the family and his socioeconomic achievements have, of course, been documented widely in other works (e.g., Strodtbeck, 1958; Blood & Wolfe, 1960; Bronfenbrenner, 1961).

MOTHER-CHILD BEHAVIOR

Mother→Child

Mother reports joint recreation, playing games, sharing mutually enjoyable activities	Mid > Lo	$p < .05$
Mother reports child does household chores	Lo > Mid	$p < .01$
Mother reports use of legitimate, referent, personalized influence techniques	Lo > Mid	$p < .01$
Mother reports anger, yelling, hitting, scolding	Lo > Hi	$p < .05$
	Lo > Mid	$p < .05$

The significant items of mother-child relationships in the SEL comparisons focus on the Lo SEL mother. All are assumed to be related to the economic and emotional pressures of being the single parent or, in the other instances, of having a passive, nonassertive husband. In both circumstances limited time and resources would interfere with the mothers' joint recreation with the children, whereas the middle-class mother was closely involved with her child. (A stereotype suggests she is sometimes too involved with him.) The Lo SEL mother often put the child into a helping role around the house. In her disciplinary efforts she reflected her restricted resources and power, appealing to the child to do what she asked as a means of being kind, good, and helpful to her. When the child would not or could not respond as she requested, the mother's frustration was often expressed in anger. The Lo SEL mother's pattern is thus similar to that exemplified by both referred father and referred mother groups. The repeated implication for Lo SEL mothers is of an interaction between relatively low levels of personal resources with high levels of economic and social pressure.

Child→Mother

Mother reports that child is responsible, does chores without urging, etc.	Hi > Lo Mid > Lo	$p < .01$ $p < .05$
Mother describes child as autonomous, independent, making his own decisions	Hi > Lo Mid > Lo	$p < .01$ $p < .05$
Mother describes child as having friends, being busy and not alone	Lo > Hi Lo > Mid	$p < .05$ $p < .05$
Mother describes child as being manipulative, performing on a contingent basis	Lo > Hi Lo > Mid	$p < .01$ $p < .01$
Mother sees child as dependent, seeking reassurance	Mid > Lo	$p < .05$

As compared to higher SEL mothers, Lo SEL mothers saw the child as requiring much urging and monitoring to carry out his responsibilities and chores. This finding may be due to SEL variations in parental control methods, the need to have children help more in Lo SEL homes (because of the absence of the father or economic pressures), or possibly the Lo SEL mother's feeling of sole responsibility for the child, which leads her to "track" him more closely. On whatever basis, our findings support the considerable literature which describes the Lo SEL mother's prevalent efforts to restrict and control her child's behavior (e.g., Waters & Crandall, 1964). As a consequence, Lo SEL children make few of their own decisions in the home. This result is not due to perceived interpersonal inadequacy, since Lo SEL mothers see their children as more socially effective (e.g., making friends) and as less dependent on them than do higher SEL mothers. The Lo SEL children often respond to maternal demands with attempts to manipulate, performing largely in response to concrete contingencies. This frustrates the mother's efforts but discourages dependency on her and does not seem to impair the child's social effectiveness outside the home, as the mother perceives it.

SUMMARY OF SEL COMPARISONS

The SEL findings for fathers emphasize differences between the extreme groups (Hi and Lo). Lo SEL fathers, when present in the home, exerted little influence on either wife or child, whereas Hi SEL fathers were central figures of interpersonal influence for their children. The largely single-parent Lo SEL mothers were different from both the Mid and Hi SEL mother groups. They saw their children as largely irresponsible but not dependent on themselves. They kept close track of their children, and their attempts at influence and control fluctuated over the total power spectrum. Hi and Mid SEL mothers described relatively responsible and autonomous children and did not seem involved in questions of responsibility or problems of control.

Referral Category Comparisons

Of the referred fathers who completed Parent Behavior Inventories, only three had aggressive (Ag) and two had hyperactive (Hy) children. Comparisons involving both these categories were therefore dropped from the analyses. Seven fathers of socially withdrawn (SW) children and 16 fathers of children with attention problems (AC) completed their forms. Mothers had seven children in each of the three categories (Ag, Hy, and SW) and 19 in AC.

A simple analysis of variance for each factor yielded few main effects for children's referral categories. Individual t tests were computed for F tests that reached the $p < .1$ level. Because of the small N's involved, most inferences derived from these data are highly tentative. Some significant indices may well be the result of chance fluctuations occurring within the large number of comparisons studied.

ATTENTION CONTROL

Parent→Spouse Behavior

Father reports wife makes decisions about money, friends, and children alone; father volunteers in community groups $AC > SW$ $p < .01$

Mother reports final decision left to father; mother is active in community groups $AC > Ag$ $p < .01$

Mother reports using personalized influence (nagging, asking favors, feeling hurt) $AC > Ag$ $p < .01$

Mother reports church and home activities for her husband $AC > SW$ $p < .05$

Attention control difficulties in children's school behavior may be related to a wide range of parental activities that take place mainly outside the home. Relative to Ag and SW groups, both parents state that the spouse makes decisions alone and both describe their own investment in community activities. These results may imply a void in parental involvement at home, with little structure being provided for the child.

Parent→Child Behavior

Father punishes child's aggressive behavior;
stops fights   AC > SW $p < .01$

Father uses personalized influence; asks child
to perform for his sake, etc.   AC > SW $p < .05$

Fathers whose children have attention control problems may deal with them in both active and passive ways. They appear to demonstrate direct action and power in order to stop the child's own assertive activity (fights), but they are low-key and indirect in exerting other kinds of influence. Alternatively, since fathers of AC children are compared here with fathers of socially inhibited children, the responses may reflect the fact that shy, withdrawing children don't require much discipline. This interpretation seems less apt if the next comparison is not a chance result: the SW child's father describes his child as more likely to be earning money, making friends easily (AC < SW, $p < .05$). This would suggest that the SW group, in situations of their own choosing, may show some initiative but in socially approved ways (relative to AC children).

A comparison (Hy < AC, $p < .05$) on a factor indicating that mothers of distractible children feel they know their child well, and know what he is feeling and doing, receives no substantiation from other data and therefore no interpretation.

SOCIAL WITHDRAWAL

Parent→Spouse Behavior

Mother reports shared decisions and activities SW > Hy $p < .05$

Mother describes father as active in household
chores   SW > Hy $p < .01$

These two factors reflect an active, amicable interaction between parents that is reminiscent of control parent responses. There is no indication of conflict. However, it may be noteworthy that the significant comparisons regarding marital interactions appear only in mother's responses. Results in data presented in the next chapter indicate that fathers of shy, inhibited children are not themselves interpersonally dominant. Thus these tentative findings in the PBI *may* reflect paternal submissiveness to the mother, instead of genuinely shared parental behavior.

Parent→Child Behavior

Father describes child as earning money, mak-
ing friends easily   SW > AC $p < .05$

Mother reports trusting the child, leaving him	SW > Ag	$p < .05$
free to do as he wishes, resolve own quarrels	SW > Hy	$p < .05$
	SW > AC	$p < .05$

Mother sees child as manipulative, performing
only for rewards   Hy > SW $p < .05$

These responses convey a positive picture of the socially inhibited child, in contrast to other referred groups. These are the only instances of specifically favorable evaluations indicated by referred parents throughout their inventories. In combination they suggest a relatively more benign family atmosphere among SW than among other referred families. However, it is possible that the mothers' highly trusting responses are due to the fact that socially withdrawing children are not likely to engage in socially challenging or aggressive interactions, so that the mother rarely needs to intrude. It seems a reasonable conjecture that these parents have less active or extreme bases for dissatisfaction with their children than parents of children with other forms of disturbance. They may be concerned about the child's social diffidence with peers at school, but they, as well as the teacher (see Chapter 5), regard their child as "good." It must be recalled, however, that this positive view of the socially withdrawn child was not significantly reflected in the FARS.

Aggression and Hyperactivity comparisons are based only on mothers' PBIs.

AGGRESSION

Parent→Spouse Behavior

Mother reports using personalized influence	SW > Ag	$p < .01$
(nagging, asking favors, feeling hurt)	AC > Ag	$p < .01$

Mother reports final decision left to father;
mother is active in community groups   AC > Ag $p < .01$

As compared to AC mothers, mothers of Ag children are less likely to defer to their husbands. They are similarly less likely to use appeals to their husband's indulgence or guilt than are mothers of SW children. In this sense they appear relatively strong and demanding.

Parent→Child Behavior

Mother sees child as dependent, needing reas-	Hy > Ag	$p < .01$
surance and comfort	SW > Ag	$p < .05$
	AC > Ag	$p < .05$

Mothers do not see their aggressive children as dependent, or as needing comfort or reassurance.

HYPERACTIVITY

Parent→Spouse Behavior

Mother reports shared decisions and activities	SW > Hy	$p < .05$
Mother describes father as active in household chores	SW > Hy	$p < .01$

Parent→Child Behavior

Mother reports trusting the child, leaving him free to do as he wishes, resolve own quarrels	SW > Hy	$p < .05$
Mother feels she knows child, what he is feeling and doing	Hy > AC	$p < .05$
Mother sees child as manipulative, performing only for rewards	Hy > SW	$p < .01$
Mother sees child as dependent, needing reassurance and comfort	Hy > Ag	$p < .01$

The general theme of these factors is that hyperactive children appear more immature to their mothers than do other referred children. They are dependent, not to be trusted, and operate on a concrete reward basis.

SUMMARY OF REFERRAL CATEGORY COMPARISONS

The referral category comparisons suggest some general commonalities within families which may relate to the children's predominant school problems, but these are not strong or definitive. This may be due in part to the small number of cases in some categories. However, it may also be that the history, structure, and norms within a familiar, though not always benign, family may lead to different patterns of behavior than those stimulated by the school environment. Although most parents of referred children agree with the school in seeing their children as troubled and disturbing, the specific "symptom" patterns in the home and school do not completely overlap. These home-school relationships are discussed further in the light of additional data.

Table 4 summarizes all significant findings described for this questionnaire.

Table 4a. Summary of Significant Comparisons: Parent Behavior Inventory—Father

Relation	Factor	Content	Referral Category				SEL		
			R	NR	SW	AC	Hi	Mid	Lo
			N=28	25	7	15	14	31	8
Fa → Mo		*Decision making*							
a	2	Share decisions and activities: home, children, go out	<**						
b	6	One parent decides alone; Fa volunteer group involvement				<**		<*Lo	
c	8	Wife decides disagreements; joint decisions on social activities, money							
d	1	*Conflict and influence* Hostile disagreement: uses wide range of influence techniques	>**						
e	4	*Identification with community* Likes neighborhood and neighbors	<*						

Table 4a. (Continued)

Relation	Factor	Content	Referral Category				SEL		
			R	NR	SW	AC	Hi	Mid	Lo
f	3	Church attendance; home maintenance; fixes things				<*		<*Lo	
		Household activities							
g	7	Mo household activities: wife decides on handling money, children, invite friends							
h	5	Fa household activities: housework, dishes, clean-up							
i	9	Ch household activities: housework, dishes, clean-up, cooking							
Fa → Ch									
		Warmth							
a	1	Affectionate: Fa shows affection in different ways; do things with and for each other							
		Interpersonal closeness							
b	6	Knows child: knows what							

c	3	he is doing; shares activities, teaches, jokes	<**		
d	4	Understands child: understands his feelings and thoughts; ch similar to wife	<**		
	4	Communication: child talks to father on various topics; work and play together	<*		
		Rationalized discipline and influence			
e	2	Ignores, physically isolates child as punishment	>(*)		
f	7	Punishes aggressive behavior; stops fights		<**	
g	5	Personalized, referent influence: asks child to perform for sake of parent	>(*)	<*	
h	8	Anger: yell, hits, scolds, shames	>**	<*	<*Lo
Ch → Fa					
		Instrumental effectiveness			
a	6	Task oriented, independent: does job well; social, but happy to work alone	<*		

Table 4a. (Continued)

Relation	Factor	Content	Referral Category				SEL		
			R	NR	SW	AC	Hi	Mid	Lo
b	7	Enthusiastic-responsible: shows enthusiasm, does work without being re-minded							
c	9	Autonomy, independence: child decides on friends, clothes					<*Lo	<*Lo	
		Interpersonally adaptive							
d	2	Affectionate: verbally and physically						<*Hi	<*Hi
e	8	Interpersonally responsive: reactive to both rewards and punishment	<*					<*Hi	<*Hi
f	4	Economic initiative: social adaptiveness, earns money, makes friends easily							
g	11	Activity level: athletic, noisy, talkative	<*			>*			
		Internalization							
h	12	Cries, whines, blames others, lack of autonomy	>*			>*			

80

i	1	Avoids personal confrontations; is tense, fearful, hostile, manipulative	
j	13	Plays alone; daydreams; seeks activity with father	>*
k	5	Sensitive to interpersonal ridicule and unfairness; somatic complaints	>**
		Ways of expressing hostility	
l	13	Hostile, defiant, angry, complains, fights, verbally and physically	>**
m	15	Verbal hostility to peers: threatens, quarrels	>**
n	10	Displaced aggression: happy when breaking things, taking things apart	
o	14	Resistance to parental control: performs when threatened; inconsistent rules	

(*) $p < .06$
** $p < .05$
*** $p < .01$

81

Table 4b. Summary of Significant Comparisons: Parent Behavior Inventory—Mother

Relation	Factor	Content	Referral Category						SEL		
			R	NR	Ag	Hy	SW	AC	Hi	Mid	Lo
			$N=34$	26	5	6	7	15	16	32	19
Mo → Fa		*Decision making*									
a	1	Share decisions and activities: home, children, go out	<**			<*SW			>**Lo >**Lo		
b	3	One parent decides alone: spending money, whom to invite	>**								
c	9	Final decisions left to Fa; Mo active in community groups			<*AC						
		Household activities									
d	10	Mo household activities: clean, cook, wash dishes									
e	4	Fa household activities				<**SW					
f	8	Ch household activities								<*Lo	

		Influence and conflict					
g	2	Disagreement, manipulation	>*		>**Ag >**Ag >*Lo		<*Hi <*Hi
h	7	Personalized influence: nags, asks for favors, would feel hurt			>**Ag >**Ag >*Lo		<*Hi <*Hi
		Identification with community					
i	6	Likes neighborhood and neighbors	<*		>**Lo >**Lo		
j	5	Church attendance; husband gardens		<AC			
Ch → Mo		*Instrumental effectiveness*					
a	5	Task oriented: persists at tasks and does them well	<**				
b	11	Responsible behavior: does chores, etc., without urging			>**Lo >**Lo		
c	3	Autonomy, independence: child decides on friends, clothes			>**Lo >**Lo		

Table 4b. (Continued)

Relation	Factor	Contents	Referral Category						SEL		
			R	NR	Ag	Hy	SW	AC	Hi	Mid	Lo
		Interpersonal adaptiveness									
d	2	Affectionate: child expresses liking for mother									
e	15	Reaction to rewards: praise, presents	<*								
f	7	Interpersonal activity: friends, general activity, not alone	<*						<*Lo	<*Lo	
g		Manipulative: performance contingent on rewards	>*						<**Lo	<**Lo	
		Internalization									
h	14	Fearful: shows fear, bites nails	>**		<*SW						
i	13	Interpersonal avoidance, tension: tense, somatic, sulks	>**								
j	6	Interpersonally sensitive: upset by scolding, unfairness									

			>**Ag	>**Ag	>*Ag	>*Lo
k	10	Dependency: seeks reassurance, comforting				
		Ways of expressing Hospitality				
l	1	Defiant: talks back, complains	>**			
m	8	Acting out hostility: hits, hurts others	>**			
n	9	Displaced aggression: breaks objects, plays alone				

(*) $p < .06$
* $p < .05$
** $p < .01$

CHAPTER 4

The Child in the Family: Behavior Samples

The two samples of behavior described in this chapter represent standardized situations in which aspects of family interactions were recorded. The first was an audiotaped Family Communication Task; the second was a video recording of family interactions.

FAMILY COMMUNICATION TASK*

In recent years it has become a truism to assert that problems of interpersonal relations are closely related to difficulties in communication (e.g., Bateson et al., 1956). However, it has been very difficult to assess either the process or the accuracy of interpersonal interchanges (e.g., Haley, 1964; Alkire, 1969). One purpose of the development of the Family Communication Task was to address this measurement problem. Some data collected in the project contain observations of total family behavior under minimally constrained interaction situations. The communication task was developed to assess only verbal interaction but to do so under conditions that permit more reliable intersubject comparisons. Here the parents and the target child participated in a task involving verbal descriptions of the graphic designs shown in Figure 4. The game-like nature of the apparatus and situation (microphones, control switches, etc., described in Appendix A, p. 244) were chosen to appeal to the largely male, 8–12 year old children in the sample. The task was for one person to provide a verbal description of one of the free-form designs while each of the others independently attempted to identify that design from an array of 16 such figures. All sessions were tape-recorded. The task was administered during the first visit and included parents and the target child. Family members alternated as senders and receivers of verbal descriptions of the designs, with the child as the initial

---

* Parts of these data were reported in Alkire, 1969. © 1969 by the American Psychological Association and reprinted by permission.

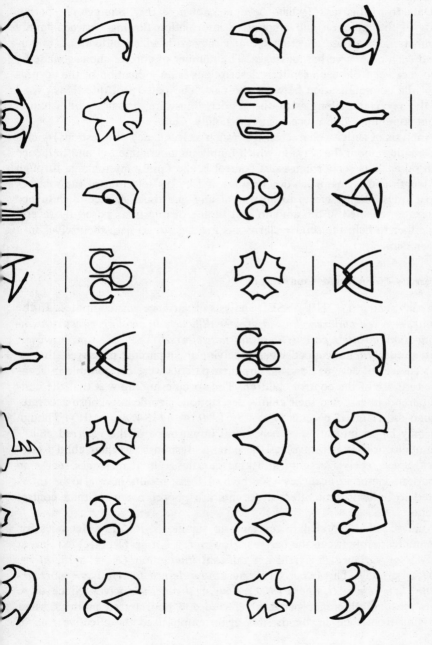

Figure 4. Designs used in Family Communications Task (the "Squiggles").

sender and each parent serving as a receiver. For single-parent families, of course, there was only one receiver.

Data from this task (which became known as the "Squiggles") permit study of the direction and amount of information flowing between family members, as well as reflecting the accuracy with which individuals understand each other's verbal messages. The number of correct choices made by each receiver from each sender's descriptions is an indication of the accuracy of the communication between the pair. The pattern of questions raised by the receivers, along with the sender's answers, provides information about communication processes in the family.

Analysis of activity characteristics (such as frequency of questions) yields information about the ways in which family members interact and influence each other. The sender can exert control in the family interchange through the length and terms of his descriptions and by his selection of the receiver whose questions he elects to answer at any one time. A second influence pattern is reflected in the amount and timing of questions posed by receivers, either to help the sender clarify his message or to help themselves in a design choice.

Referred—Nonreferred Comparisons

For each sender a R/NR × SEL analysis of variance was computed. In the results, *referred children showed greater difficulty in sending effective communications to their parents than did nonreferred.* They did not, however, seem similarly handicapped when receiving their parents messages, that is, their choices of designs described by their parents were comparable in accuracy to those of the control children. The specific finding was that the control parents interpreted their child's descriptions significantly more accurately than did referred parents ($F = 9.61$, $df = 1/134$, $p < .01$). Though this may be an indication of behavioral impairment of the referred child's communication, it also involves the parents' responses to their child's messages. Since receiver activity in asking questions about messages seems an important factor in accuracy (see below) these results may also be interpreted to indicate that referred parents are poorer receivers than control parents.

Analyses of parental data revealed no significant R/NR differences for communication between the parents. However, a Group (R, NR) × Parent analysis of variance did yield a significant interaction ($F = 5.25$, $df = 1/67$, $p < .05$). This occurred because *nonreferred fathers were more accurate than referred fathers when receiving from their wives.* Since there was almost no difference between referred and nonreferred mothers when receiving from their husbands, this again emphasized the effective role of the nonreferred father in interaction with his wife. However, further evidence was needed to indicate whether the control father's role in the family was also the decisive factor in the initial finding that control parents interpret their children's messages more accurately than referred parents.

Previous studies with this task had indicated that accuracy was related strongly to the amount of clarifying questions asked of the sender, that is, to the activity of the receiver (Alkire, Collum, Kaswan, & Love, 1968; Alkire, 1970). Preliminary analysis of questioning behavior in this study revealed that *in the nonreferred group, the father asked the first question of the child twice as often as the mother* ($F = 5.44$, $df = 1/27$, $p < .05$). Usually the nonreferred father then continued to ask for clarification until he made his choice. In these cases the mother generally asked no question until the father was finished. This pattern is reminiscent of the paradigm for effective leadership in families described by Murrell and Stachowiak (1967), in which one parent is supported in a clear leadership role by the spouse.

In the referred group, mothers and fathers were about equal in frequency of first interventions and they interrupted each other much more than did nonreferred parents. This lack of role structure and/or interpersonal consideration between referred parents appears many times in our measures, most notably in PBI influence patterns. Similarly, the interpersonal activity demonstrated in the control fathers' questions supports the positive, active involvement he described for himself in his Inventory responses, along with his clearly established influence over his child. It further substantiated the highly positive social impact attributed to him by his spouse and child on the adjective ratings.

The content of messages and amount of questions between parents have not as yet been analyzed. It is not known, therefore, whether the higher accuracy of nonreferred fathers noted above is due to the clarity of their wives' messages, the result of the husbands' questioning, or some combination of the two. The general finding goes along with the mutual discussion and decision-making pattern claimed by both control parents on their behavior questionnaires. As such, it may reflect practice effects.

For whatever reasons, including the evidence for the basic role of the father in eliciting and evoking higher quality of responses, referred children seem to send poorer messages than the controls. This point was given some additional support in a supplementary study in which college students were given both referred and nonreferred children's initial descriptions of each design. They made more accurate choices of designs from the messages of the nonreferred children, as parents had done. It would seem that more intensive investigation of the informational content of communications from troubled children may help clarify the relationship between communication and interpersonal difficulties.

To illustrate the contrast between children's effective and ineffective communication to parents, examples from referred and control cases are presented below.

The child in the first example was a 9 year old girl, painfully shy and dependent, extremely overprotected and overcontrolled by the mother (referral category III, Social Withdrawal, high severity). She had no known social interactions with other children and was failing the second grade for the second time although she was of average intelligence. The single-parent mother had few if any social contacts outside the home so that almost the only meaningful interactions this mother and child had were with each other. Their total interaction for this design was as follows:

Ch: Well, this one has a very *funny* design on it and it's a little bit going in and out.
Mo: What kind of a design would you say it was, dear?
Ch: Well, it's—a very *funny* design and it's almost like a leaf on a tree.
Mo: Um-hum, that's fine—all right.

Clearly, the description is not very informative—the child described almost all of the designs as "a leaf." The mother's questions did not help much and although this choice, as well as almost all the other choices the mother made, was in error, she seemed satisfied.

By contrast, two examples of control children's interactions with their father seem to epitomize the differences we have been describing.

1. Ch: Well, it looks like a, a bat . . . a batman's ring and its got 5 points and . . . um . . .
   Fa: Johnny?
   Ch: Yeah?
   Fa: Does it look like a king's crown?
   Ch: Yes, in a way.
   Fa: And you had it (the design) before?
   Ch: Yes.
   Fa: Thank you.

2. Ch: Oh, no, not this one! . . . Like the moon . . . a backwards moon.
   Fa: What did you say it looked like, Dave?
   Ch: A backwards moon . . .
   Fa: Ah, does it have a . . . look like a L shape . . . backwards?
   Ch: Yeah . . .
   Fa: Does it have a little ditch on the bottom of it where the arm comes out? . . . a little . . .
   Ch: What?

Fa: Does it have a little dip on the bottom of it . . . where the . . . on the L?
Ch: Yeah.
Fa: Just a little dip down there?
Ch: Yeah . . .
Fa: Okay, thank you . . .
Ch: Signing off.
Fa: Over and out.

The protective, vague, bland terms in which the referred mother evaded the task for both herself and her daughter stand in marked contrast to the specific concepts contributed by the control fathers. The first stance is as passive and ineffectual as the second is active, productive, and indicative of mutual enjoyment.

The differences in the quality of messages between nonreferred and referred families appear to be quite consistent and are generally independent of measured intelligence (Alkire, 1967).

Socioeconomic Level Comparisons

A relationship was found between accuracy of design choice and SEL ($F =$ 3.49, $df = 2/134$, $p < .05$). *The SEL effect is most regular and striking in communications between the parents, showing a linear decrease of accuracy in parental communication in the order of Hi > Mid > Lo SEL in both the father-to-mother and mother-to-father combinations.* Though the number of cases in the Hi and Lo SEL groups is small, the replication of this effect in referred and nonreferred groups provides some weight for the finding. The relatively poor accuracy of the Lo groups is probably best explained by the more limited range of verbal communication reported widely for lower class groups (Eiduson, 1968). We have not as yet analyzed in detail the language patterns used by different SEL groups in this task, but preliminary tabulations do indicate briefer messages and less receiver questioning in Lo than in Mid or Hi SEL groups. The slight, but consistently poorer accuracy of the Mid relative to the Hi SEL group repeats the linear relationship between Ammons' IQ and SEL described in Chapter 2.

There were no (R, NR) × SEL interaction trends of even borderline significance, indicating that this effect is not confounded with the troubled behavior of the referred families.

Referral Category Comparisons

In Referral Category × Receiver analysis of variance for each sender, the analysis for the mother showed a main category effect tending toward significance ($F = 2.38$, $df = 3/40$, $p < .10$). The same rank order of accuracy appeared in the different referral categories in the mother-to-father and mother-to-child combinations: Aggression > Attention Control > Social Withdrawal > Hyperactivity. This rank order is also essentially replicated by the dyadic mother sending to the child (only two dyad children were classified as predominantly socially withdrawn and therefore are not counted here). The tendency of mothers of aggressive children to use direct, active verbal styles was indicated in the PBIs. This characteristic might be expected to contribute to accuracy since success in the task depends, in part, on an active question-answer relationship.

Other referral category differences in accuracy have not been analyzed further because of the small number of cases in the Hyperactivity and Social Withdrawal categories.

Summary

Children in referred families were found to send poorer verbal descriptions of graphic designs than children in nonreferred families. Control group fathers took a more active and constructive role in questioning their children than did the referred fathers, and they were more accurate than referred fathers when receiving from their wives. Accuracy of parents' choices varied directly with SEL in the order of Hi > Mid > Lo. With respect to the child's predominant referral category, there was a trend indicating that with mother as sender to either the father or child, accuracy of receivers' choices was in the order Aggression > Attention Control > Social Withdrawal > Hyperactivity.

The most interesting finding is probably that nonreferred fathers were more accurate than referred fathers when receiving from mothers. This further substantiates the consistent pattern of results from other measures, again showing the nonreferred father's more effective behavior with his wife as well as with his child.

VIDEOTAPES OF FAMILY INTERACTIONS

Each family was observed and videotaped at the outset of their first appointment in the clinic. A number of precautions had been taken to ensure that parents knew of these procedures in advance and had had an opportunity to express any objections, questions, or concerns that might arise. As soon as an initial appointment was scheduled a standard letter went out to the family. This described training and research functions of the clinic which necessitated observation and recording as part of our efforts to improve our services and develop new ways of working with people's problems. The letter gave names and telephone numbers of staff for parents to call if they wished to ask questions about any clinic procedures. The day before the scheduled intake appointment, the project secretary telephoned the family to confirm both the appointment and the family's receipt of the letter. If there seemed to be any hesitation with respect to the letter, or if any question was raised about clinic procedures, the secretary transferred the call to one of the project directors. This happened in only two or three instances. After discussion of our policies about observation and recording, we offered referral to other facilities, should the parents still feel at all hesitant about our procedures. In each instance, however, the parents elected to keep their original appointment.

In a few cases, numerous attempts to reach a family by phone on the day before their appointment were unsuccessful. For these, the secretary checked the family case folder to be sure that the carbon of the standard letter was there, that the date on it indicated that there had been adequate time for delivery of the letter. When the family arrived for the appointment, she determined that the letter had indeed been received.

The family was shown into the clinic "family" room which had a standard arrangement of furniture and supplies, including toys and refreshments (but no reading material). They were told that a clinician would join the family in a few minutes. A one-way vision screen covered most of one wall and a microphone hung from the ceiling in the middle of the room. A video camera behind the screen was barely visible but was often spotted by the families. Videotaping began when the family entered and was continuous throughout a standard sequence of interactions covering a period of 15–25 minutes (depending upon family size).

The unstructured nature of the situation, along with the clear indications of observation and recording, put all families under some degree of self-consciousness or apprehension. Reactions varied widely, from nervousness and joking to suspicion and anger, veiled or overt. In this setting, parents set widely varying limits for their children and showed different degrees of personal and interpersonal protective concern. Verbal and nonverbal activity reflected alignments, exclusions, overtures, and withdrawals in parental, parent-child, and sibling patterns. The wide range of behaviors manifested, even under these observed conditions, show that the videotapes reflected diversified, if sometimes constrained, examples of familial interactions. Observation clearly affected the families' behavior, but it appeared that reactions to the strange setting included behavior peculiar to each family's pattern for dealing with stress.

The first 5 minutes of the videotape was a period of "free" interaction during which there was no external structure of activity provided for the family. They were waiting: for an unspecified period of time, for an unknown clinician, and for an undefined experience. After 5 minutes, the clinician entered and met the family. A sequence of arrangements followed during which the interactions of mother-child, father-child, and mother-father were recorded, each for about 3 minute periods. This sequential arrangement permitted the sampling of interactions in the different combinations of the basic family triad. (Details of these arrangements are described in Appendix A, pp. 246–247.)

The total family was then reassembled in the family room and asked to spend a few minutes discussing each person's understanding of why they had come to the clinic and what each person would like to have changed in their family. This request was given in a relatively standard (though not verbatim) text. Five minutes of the ensuing discussion among family members, termed the "Problem Definition," constituted the end of the videotaped interaction.

An intrinsic problem in comparing referred and nonreferred family patterns was, as always, the difference in the motives of the two groups for being present in the clinic. In seeking to make the most valid comparisons possible, we tried to identify the situations which would be most similar for both groups. In pilot studies we had observed that all families upon first entering the family room seemed to respond to the refreshments, toys, blackboard, seating arrangements, microphone, and one-way vision screen. On this basis we assumed that these initially salient characteristics of the setting would make the first few moments our most equivalent context for both sets of families; the attention of all seemed focused on the external situation. Therefore our initial group comparisons were limited to the first 5 minutes of the observed situation, although ratings made of the entire tapes are also reported. We had anticipated that differences would become greater during later periods. For example, communication seemed likely to become much more negative among referred families during the problem definition period, when they talked about their current problems, than among control families who presumably had no besetting difficulties to consider.

These videotapes have been analyzed in several ways. Repeated viewing of discrete segments of tape, made possible by the video recorder's playback capability, yield fine-grained analyses of behavior which add depth and specificity to the patterns of family interaction under study. Descriptions of two analyses are included here.*

* Portions of these results are also reported in Bugental, Love, Kaswan, and April, 1971, and Bugental, Love, and Kaswan, 1972. © 1971 and © 1972 by the American Psychological Association and reprinted by permission.

Study I: Evaluative, Activity, and Directing Components of Family Behavior

This analysis focused on the evaluative, activity, and influencing characteristics of the verbal and nonverbal behavior of parents and the target child (referred or control) as video recorded during their initial appointment. Ratings were made of each member of the triad in terms of the three interpersonal dimensions for each successive 30 second section of the family videotapes. The goal was to determine whether there were discriminable differences in these behavioral characteristics between the two groups of families.

Since the rating process involved was very time consuming, this detailed analysis was limited to 20 referred and 10 nonreferred family tapes. The two subsets of families were matched for socioeconomic level and sex of child. Beyond this, families were chosen only in terms of the technical quality of their videotapes. Appendix B, Table 7 provides information on the characteristics of the subsample. The only significant difference in background between referred and nonreferred groups was in family composition. Nine out of 20 referred families contained only one parent, whereas all non-referreds contained two parents. This difference reflected the general high incidence of broken homes in the background of the referred children (see Chapter 2).

RATING PROCEDURES

During a rating session two judges were shown one videotape at a time. The video recorder was stopped every 30 seconds and ratings were made of one person on each of three dimensions.

Ratings were based on the rater's immediate impression of verbal *and* nonverbal behavior. The three dimensions, high to low activity, high to low directiveness, and positive to negative evaluation, were defined for the raters by repeated showing of videotaped scenes of actors portraying typical family roles. These scenes had been constructed to include examples of high and low levels of each dimension as they were demonstrated in each of the three components of interpersonal messages, the visual, vocal, and verbal. (The high and low levels of the dimensions in the scenes had been established by other judges).* Raters were asked to use these polar scenes as anchors for their ratings but brief additional verbal descriptions of the dimensions were also provided:

1. Activity: the amount of energy expended in a communication.

---

* See Bugental et al. (1971) for further details.

2. Directing, or influencing: the extent to which a communication explicitly attempts to direct or limit the behavior of another person.

3. Positive versus negative evaluation: the extent to which a communication is friendly, approving, and considerate, rather than unfriendly, disapproving, or inconsiderate.

The three sets of scores were obtained from ratings of the total behavior of each family member for each successive 30 second time period of the videotape. Raters were instructed to focus on one person's behavior during each tape segment and to ignore, as much as possible, behavior in previous sections or the behavior of other people, including their reactions to the person being rated. In this way we maintained our focus on a particular person's behavior, rather than on interactions, in order to permit more direct comparison with our other data. Presumably the instructions to raters would minimize, though not wholly eliminate, the impact of the interpersonal context within each message and the influence of preceding periods.

The activity and directing dimensions were rated on a scale from 0 to 6. The evaluative dimension was rated on a scale from $+6$ to -6 with a midpoint at zero. These three primary dimensions were not correlated strongly in any consistent way (Appendix B, Table 8).

A supplementary measure was the amount of time each member of the family talked, as measured with a stopwatch. Interjudge agreement among two judges was high (r fathers $= +.95$; r children $= +.96$). Since amount of talking had been used as an index of dominance or control by others (e.g., Farina, 1960; Hetherington, 1967), we could examine the relations between this measure and our independent assessments of attempts at interpersonal influence, that is, ratings made of his directiveness. Also we could compare judgments of a person's general activity with the measured amount of his talking. When amount of talking was demonstrated to be relatively independent of the other dimensions (Appendix B, Table 9) it was included as an additional (fourth) variable. (It was later reanalyzed as a covariate, as will be described.)

RATERS

The raters were five parent-aged women drawn from a larger pool of project raters. They were trained for approximately 4 hours by making repeated ratings of practice videotaped scenes and receiving feedback on previous ratings made by others. Interjudge agreement was measured on the basis of their ratings of actual family tapes subsequent to preliminary selection and training procedures. The median interjudge reliabilities (r) for ratings of activity were $+.80$, $+.64$, and $+.84$ (mother, father, child); $+.85$, $+.71$, and $+.76$ for ratings of directing; and $+.81$, $+.90$, and $+.71$ for ratings of positive to negative qualities of behavior. These reliabilities are not uniformly high but, with the exception of father-activity ratings, are considered acceptable. The judges were unaware of the purpose of the project and had no other information about the families. None of the judges had a background in psychology. There is evidence from other research that naive judges can make global ratings of this kind as reliably and validly as experienced judges (Shapiro, 1968). Indeed, we feel that the interrater agreement obtained by unsophisticated judges with the brief training provided indicates that the scales had considerable face validity.

RESULTS

Raters' scores of the 30 tapes revealed that mothers as a group were seen as more directing and talkative than fathers (Appendix B, Table 10). On the positive to negative dimension, although there were no differences for mean ratings between parent groups, mothers were rated as showing more extreme behaviors on this affective-expressive dimension than were fathers. Such maternal extremes were sometimes positive (the mothers were rated as being highly friendly and approving) or sometimes negative (they seemed highly disapproving and inconsiderate); sometimes they were seen in sequences of both extremes, suggesting an emotionally charged atmosphere in which much approval and/or disapproval was being expressed. This observed variability was reflected most aptly in the range of ratings assigned to each individual on the positive to negative evaluation dimension.* The preponderance of these extreme ratings of expressive behavior given to the mothers was quite consistent though the group (mother versus father) comparisons did not achieve levels of statistical significance. This directive, talkative, affectively toned pattern replicates an earlier finding (Merrill, 1946): mothers tend to demonstrate controlling and intrusive behavior when they and their children are being observed, in an apparent effort to elicit socially desirable behavior from the children.

Referred-Nonreferred Comparisons. There were no significant differences between referred and nonreferred mothers in the raters' judgments on any of the three dimensions. Because of the significant role generally assigned to mothers' behavior for children's developmental characteristics, this finding was quite unexpected. It seems most likely due to the generalized effect of the observed clinic situation. All mothers seemed to have the com-

---

* Not only were group differences for this characteristic slightly more significant for range than for variance, the evaluative behavior was more typically characterized by expression of extremes (often only a single incident, either highly positive or highly negative) rather than by affective lability, that is, shifting back and forth from positive to negative affect.

mon reactions described above and expressed them in somewhat comparable ways, at least in such superficial matters as supervising coat removal, seating, snacks, and use of play materials.

As with most of our findings, the most consistent differences between referred and nonreferred families involved the fathers (see Appendix B, Table 10). *Referred fathers were more directive (p < .05) and more talkative (p < .05) than control fathers; they also received extreme ratings for expressive behavior, either positive or negative (R > NR, p < .01). Thus the behavior of referred fathers was rated as being very similar to that of the total mother group (referred and nonreferred): they were highly directive of the child's actions, talked a lot, and frequently expressed extreme approval or disapproval. In contrast, the fathers of nonreferred children could be described as "low-key" in interactions with their families.* They rarely became ruffled; they talked little and gave few directions; their comments were in large measure devoid of approval or disapproval. Anecdotally, the overall impression given by these fathers was that they were relatively relaxed and self-confident. The contrast between father groups is best described by the "anxious emotional involvement" versus "calm detachment" differentiation made by Becker (1964).

Although there were too few girls in our sample for meaningful statistical comparisons, the differences between fathers of referred and nonreferred girls were of the same magnitude and direction as differences between fathers of boys.

In a reanalysis of these data, the amount of talking was treated as a covariate (Bugental et al., 1972). It became clear that some referred fathers tended to be highly verbal whereas others spoke very little. Thus in contrast to control fathers who were low on all three variables (directiveness, talkativeness, and display of evaluative affect), referred fathers displayed both directiveness and high levels of affect, but could be either high or low on talkativeness. The differential relationships of the two referred father patterns with their children's behavior are described later, in the referral category comparisons.

Referred and nonreferred children were also significantly different from each other in the ratings they received on the positive to negative dimension. *Referred children, like their fathers, demonstrated greater expressive extremes than did nonreferred children (p < .01).* Again, the same trend was found for boys and girls.

These differences between referred and control families were derived from the scores for the first 5 minute segments of the family videotape, but contrary to expectation, initial differences were maintained across all time periods. Referred fathers were more directing (see Figure 5) and more talkative (Figure 6) throughout the entire videotape.

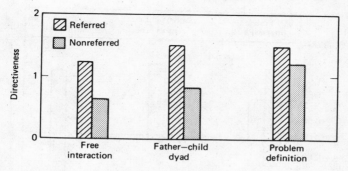

Figure 5. *Father directing*: a mixed-design analysis of variance containing one between-subjects variable (group) and one within-subjects variable (time) produced a significant main effect for groups ($F = 8.16$; $df = 1, 19$; $p < .05$).

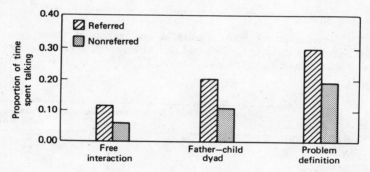

Figure 6. *Father talking*: a mixed-design analysis of variance containing one between-subjects (group) and one within-subjects variable (time) produced a trend for group differences ($F = 3.59$; $df = 1, 19$; $p = .10$).

Referred fathers (see Figure 7) and referred children (see Figure 8) received ratings at both extremes of the evaluative dimension across all time periods. Sometimes the large evaluative ranges reflected higher positive extremes, sometimes higher negative extremes, and sometimes both, but the total evaluative range was consistently greater for ratings of these fathers and children over all time periods. It would seem on this basis that the differential behavior patterns show a fair degree of generality.

The high directiveness found to be typical of referred fathers has been observed previously in conjunction with childhood adjustment problems. Peterson et al., (1959), for example, found that the parents of children seen at a guidance clinic with problems similar to those of ours were low on "democratic guidance" in comparison with the parents of nonclinic children. Also, the fathers of clinic children made more suggestions to their children than

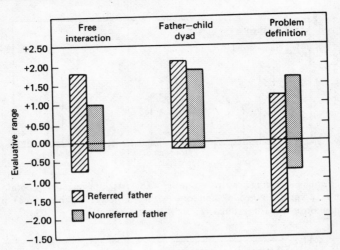

Figure 7. *Father evaluative range:* a mixed-design analysis of variance containing one between-subjects variable (group) and one within-subjects variable (time) produced a significant main effect for groups ($F = 5.08$; $df = 1, 19$; $p < .05$).

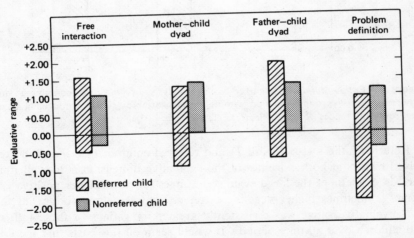

Figure 8. *Child evaluative range:* a mixed-design analysis of variance containing one between-subjects variable (group) and one within-subjects variable (time) produced a significant main effect for groups ($F = 11.46$; $df = 1, 19$; $p < .01$).

nonclinic fathers. In our data it is important to note that reference is being made to fathers' *effort at directing* the child's behavior, *not to the success or effectiveness of these efforts.* We focused here, as elsewhere in the study, on the behaviors of individuals, not their interactions.

The extremely evaluative (or affective) behavior attributed to fathers and mothers, coupled with high directiveness by both parents, made a distinct pattern of parental behavior in referred families. The children were continuously groomed, criticized, offered food, encouraged, instructed, teased, restrained, and watched by both parents. In nonreferred families this role was characteristic only of mothers.

The pattern of paternal extremes of expressiveness, combined with directiveness and talkativeness, is illustrated by excerpts from two referred families. The referred child in the first example, a 9 year old girl, was described as hyperactive, extremely withdrawn, dependent, socially isolated, and distractible. The following segment is drawn from the problem definition period. During this interaction two brothers (preschool and first grade) were being physically restrained by the parents at one side of the room and the target child was sitting opposite. The father's voice was condescendingly positive throughout this excerpt.

Father: Now you listen to me and let's see if you understand me.
[overlapping] If you don't . . . when you're done, you . . .
Sib 1:   . . . I want to go back in there.
Father: You listen to me though and if you don't understand me you tell me to explain it to you, all right? Dr. Love wants us to . . . listen to me . . . look at me and listen to me,
[overlapping] all right, she wants us to tell what we can do to help make ourselves better and why are we here . . . you know why we're here Ricky?
Mother: . . . an ahh . . .
Sib 1:   [mumbles] . . .
Mother: [to Sib 1]: . . . or do you want to change somebody else? Do you want to change somebody in this family? . . .
[overlapping]
Sib 1:   . . . [mumbles] . . .
Sib 2:   I don't know why we're here . . .
Mother: Do you want to change somebody in the family . . . do you want to change or don't you want to change?
[overlapping]
Sib 1:   [mumble, cranky cry] . . .
Child: . . . Another family . . . can we change us to another family?
Father: No, how we can change . . . You are interrupting young man . . . You are interrupting . . . his eyes are crusty again, by the way . . .
[overlapping]
Sib 1:   . . . Daddy, what can I play with?

Mother:　. . . you broke it, now it's just too bad. I told you not to pour it . . .

Father:　What we can do . . . what are we going to do . . . to help change ourselves and change . . . ourselves . . .

[overlapping]

Mother:　. . . keep it . . . keep it on one subject [to father] . . . stop it . . . [to child].

Father:　and somebody, someone else in our family so that we will have a nicer family life.

The second example is drawn from a family in which both children were described as having problems in school, although the girl was the referred case. She was reported by her teachers to have difficulty in paying attention and concentrating on her schoolwork, and to have very poor relations with other children, appearing exceedingly shy and withdrawn. The boy, on the other hand, was described as aggressive and disruptive in his relationships with schoolmates. The father's behavior in the family room was rated as directive, talkative, and extremely negative. The following conversation occurred during the problem definition period.

Mother:　Well, now Kathy came home from school today and said that the teacher had bawled her out for saying shut up. Who she's saying this is this one kid—this Ellen Tate—that teases Kathy all the time, and I told Kathy that I think she should mention it to the . . .

Boy
[interrupting]:　Hey, man, they really do have a microphone (father had initially pointed out the possibility of TV cameras to the boy).

Father:　Yeah, yeah, now take it easy.

Boy:　It works, too.

Father:　Yeah, I know, but your mother's talking, Bobby. What were you saying, darling [turning to mother].

Mother:　That she has to tell . . .

Boy:　[additional undecipherable comment]

Mother:　Be quiet!

Father:　Your mother is speaking. Now what is it?

[Mother and child both start to talk again]

Father:　[yelling] Bobby, I'm going to slap you right across the mouth.

Mother:　Now sit down.

Father:　[still yelling] Now, is that clear? Now, come over here and sit down. Come on, sit down . . . Now, darling, what was it [turning to mother].

Mother: I think Mrs. Cleaver should know that Ellen Tate is irritating Kathy into this business of saying "shut up."

Father: Right. I do, too.

[to girl] You're going to have to learn eventually to just ignore such things . . . because the more they make you angry, or they think that you get angry, the more they're going to keep going at it as long as you keep showing that you're angry. Now you may be angry at them but you don't say anything. You just ignore them . . . you don't say anything.

This father demonstrated marked inconsistency—reacting in an explosively negative fashion one minute and recommending restraint of anger the next. Such incongruences suggest the extent to which parents are often unaware of the content and contradictions in their own communication patterns.

The father's behavior was frequently mirrored in the child's behavior. The correlations between the father's and the child's behavior are significant on all three dimensions found to distinguish referred and nonreferred families (Appendix B, Table 11). Talkative fathers tended to have talkative children ($r = .41$, $p < .05$); directive fathers had directive children ($r = .45$, $p < .05$); fathers given extreme ratings on the evaluative dimension had children whose ratings were comparably extreme ($r = .78$, $p < .01$). (Correlations between ratings given mothers and their children in the family room were consistently nonsignificant except for an inverse relationship on activity.) These relationships suggest the possibility of a modeling process, although it may be equally valid to suppose that the father's behavior is responsive to that of his child. The close relationship between father and child behavior in the videotaped interactions repeats the reported similarities described in the adjective ratings and the behavior inventories.

These observations hold only when the father and child are together in the family room. They cannot be generalized directly to the school situation where, as we shall see, the behavior of the child may be quite different from that shown in interaction with his family. There were too few girls in our sample to draw any firm conclusions about the relationship between sex of child and child-father similarity in behavior. However, there were indications that this was as great for girls as for boys, since the rank-order correlation between the evaluative range of girls ($n = 5$) and the evaluative range of their fathers was $+ .93$ ($p < .05$).

Socioeconomic Level Comparisons. The small number of control families in this subsample made meaningful SEL comparisons impossible, especially with respect to behavior of fathers. It would appear, however, that the directing, talkative, highly affective behavior of the referred fathers was limited largely to middle-class fathers. Our impression of *all* the families seen (not just those subjected to detailed analysis) was that referred lower-class fathers (most of whom were black) were characterized by low interaction of any type with their family. This is supported by results of Parent Behavior Inventory SEL analyses which indicated a consistently low activity, low power role for these fathers.

Referral Category Comparisons. Comparisons were made within the referred sample on the basis of type and severity of the child's referral problem. Separate correlations were computed between severity scores for children classified in each referral category and ratings on all dimensions (Apppendix B, Table 12). In addition to the results of these correlational analyses, findings are included which were based upon the reanalyses of the original data using analysis of covariance techniques, with amount of talking as the covariate (Bugental et al., 1972). In these analyses the original directive, talkative, and affective behavior described for referred fathers as a group proved to be characteristic only of fathers of aggressive and distractible children. Fathers of withdrawn children were significantly distinguished from fathers of nonreferred children only on the basis of their high levels of verbalization.

In terms of these analyses, behaviors in the clinic that seem associated with children's problems in school are considered for the four categories in turn.

Aggressive Behavior. The severity of the aggressive behavior attributed to the child in school was found to be significantly correlated with the ratings given the father's behavior in the family room on two dimensions: his directiveness, and his expression of negative affect. Relationships between severity of child aggressiveness with the evaluative dimension were in fact significant for *(a)* the average rating given the father on the evaluative dimension $(r = +.65)$, *(b)* the ratings made of his positive behavior $(r = +.55)$, and *(c)* the ratings made of his negative extremes of expressive behavior $(r = +.77)$. *The more disapproving, unfriendly, or inconsiderate the father in the family room and the more directive his behavior, the more likely the child to have received high severity scores on aggressiveness in school.* However, there was no correlation between father negativity and child negativity in their interactions $(r = -.02)$. It appears that when the father is highly negative, the child is likely to act out hostile behavior in the school where it may be less dangerous than with his highly reactive parent.

This father-child relationship may be interpreted either in a modeling framework or in some version of the frustration-aggression hypothesis. The modeling hypothesis would assure that the children copy the father's behavior but only when they are in the relatively safe school environment or some other remote situation. The frustration-aggression hypothesis would suggest that the repressive environment at home creates a great deal of frustration which stimulates aggressive behavior at school.

These findings are consistent with (though not identical to) the results of other investigators who have found that regardless of socioeconomic level or method of study, aggressive boys come from homes in which parents are rejecting and punitive (e.g., Bandura & Walters, 1959; McCord et al., 1961; Sears et al., 1953). Although a number of families in this study could be described in these terms, others did not appear to behave with the negative intent or extremes implied in such adjectives. With ratings of more extremely antisocial, acting out children than those still being maintained within the public school system, more extremely negative paternal behaviors might well be involved.

The following interaction, which occurred in the family of a boy with predominantly aggressive problems in school, gives a feeling for the behavior of this type of father. The exchange came after a discussion about the mother's working. The mother had just scolded the girl for giggling.

Mother: This is very serious, Lisa, we're taking people's time . . .
[interrupting]:
Girl I . . . I stopped laughing.
Girl: I . . .
[simultaneously]
Boy: I can't eat.
Girl: I'm going to the bathroom, is that all right?
Mother: No, sit down.
Mother: Alan, turn, go sit over there where she doesn't have to look at you.
Father: Swell, isn't it?
[Girl turns away, puts face in hand to hide smile.]
Mother: Alan, what about when I do come home after school?
Father Lisa, I'm going to get up and I'm going to break your so-
[interrupting]: and-so neck.
Mother: They're listening to you.
Father: I don't give a damn.
Mother: They're recording everything you say.
Father: Good! Maybe they'll know the truth.

The mother's voice in the preceding interaction was consistently soft, saccharine, and whiny. The father's voice was abrupt and loud. The boy was typically pleasant and friendly, and he at no time expressed any anger.

Hyperactivity. None of the three dimensions measured were significantly correlated with Hyperactivity.

Social Withdrawal. There was a high correlation between severity scores on the child's socially withdrawn behavior at school and the father's talkativeness in the clinic ($r = .81$, $p < .01$). There was also a trend ($r = +.43$) for the child's talkativeness in the family room to be related to his social withdrawal at school. These relationships do not seem to fit a "dominance" interpretation of talkativeness since directiveness is not high in this subgroup of fathers (Appendix B, Table 12). If referred fathers and children talk because they are nervous or fearful, the child's behavior can be understood as one of modeling. Also in the family room where these interactions occurred, fathers' questioning of children required responses from them. Much of these children's talking was of this unspontaneous nature. The most reasonable interpretation of the high verbal levels of these fathers seems to be that it represents a socially dependent response to a somewhat stressful situation. This is in line with a suggestion relating high amounts of talking under stress conditions to affiliative or situationally dependent behavior (Rabbie, 1963).

In this analysis, as with our other measures, parents whose other responses suggested personal insecurity often tended to adopt low power positions for themselves. These implicitly demanded greater responsibility, activity, self-control, or effectiveness from the child. In videotaped interactions some parents consistently directed attention and conversation to the child, as if to draw attention away from themselves. This quite obviously heightened the child's discomfort, especially since his uneasy reaction to being observed was already usually manifest. Parental attempts to reduce their own discomfort often seemed to result in increased tension for the child, though there was usually no indication that the parents either intended or noticed the consequences of their behavior for the child.

The following excerpt is from the family of a child described as withdrawn, apathetic, and socially isolated. In the family room the father was talkative and tense. During the entire interaction the father kicked one foot and his forehead was wrinkled upward, giving him a tense, worried expression.

Father: Billy, come here.
          [Father looks around room, up at the ceiling, etc.]
Father: How are your knuckles today, Bill?
          [Father picks lint off his pants.]
Sib: Fine.
Father: (to child) Get a napkin for yourself, darling.
          [points to napkin, then rests jaw in hand and rubs his face]

Father: [to child] Wipe your mouth [points to own mouth].
Sib: Do you think that Doctor's watching us?
Father: Wipe your mouth.
          [Father pulls nose over to one side of face.]
Mother: No one's watching us.
Father: No one's watching us. I'm sure they're not.
Child: I think they are.
          [Father pulls nose over again.]
Father: Take the napkin . . . there's a wastebasket over there.
Child: Where?
Father: Right in the corner.
          [Father looks at wife with faint smile, then looks at watch.]

*Attention Control. Attention Control severity ratings for the child at
school were found to be related to the father's talkativeness and to ratings of
his expressive extremes.* The greater the range of the ratings made of the
father's expressive behavior, the greater the likelihood that the child had
been described as distractible and inattentive in class ($r = .60$, $p < .05$).
Additionally, children with marked attention control problems in school
were rated as active ($r = .53$, $p < .05$) and friendly, both in terms of average evaluative content ($r = .49$, $p < .05$) and extremes of positiveness
($r = .59$, $p < .01$) in the family room. Judges, rating for small time intervals, tended to give positive ratings to "distractible" children who laughed
and smiled often while actively engaged in play. It was our impression that
longer observation of these children would be likely to lead to the judgment
that they were being "silly" or "clowning."

In order to test this possibility (that high positive ratings had been given
to small units of behavior during times when children were engaged in immature, "silly" behavior), a comparison was made of the extreme ratings
given older and younger referred and nonreferred children. In the referred
sample there were no significant age differences for behavior that was rated
as either highly positive or negative. Among the nonreferred children, 8 and
9 year olds received more extreme ratings than those aged 10 or more ($p
< .05$), with the difference being due mainly to the higher positive ratings
made of the younger nonreferred children. It seems likely therefore that
brief units of "silly" behavior may have received positive ratings.

Both distractibility and extreme ranges of affective behavior involve a
concept of fluctuation and variability (in mood, attention, and the like).
The immature, distractible, poorly motivated behavior of Attention Control
children in school may be one type of generalized response to the intrusive,
emotional behavior of their parents who in effect treat the children as if
they were much younger than their chronological age. It is indeed possible

that the referred children acted immature because they were treated as immature. This feature of parental interaction with referred children was especially apparent in the use of babyish endearments, in parental failure to consider the child's dignity, and an overall anxious concern that attributed little competence to the child.

Alternatively, it is possible that children who demonstrate a high amount of play activity in the clinic and distractibility at school may *elicit* the observed response pattern from their parents. Thus affectively labile children may constitute strong and disturbing stimuli and may induce adults to attempt to control them through relatively extreme expressions of approval and disapproval.

SUMMARY

An analysis of the first 5 minutes of unstructured videotaped family interaction revealed no differences between referred and nonreferred mothers. Behavior of referred fathers, however, was rated as more directive, more talkative, and including more instances of extremes of affect than that of nonreferred fathers. These differences were maintained throughout the recorded period. Overall, the behavior of children in the clinic was found to be highly correlated with the father's behavior in this same setting. In additional analyses, the father's family room behavior was found to be related to the type of problem the child manifested in school: (*a*) father negativity in the family room was significantly correlated with child aggressiveness at school, (*b*) father talkativeness in the clinic (seen as a socially dependent response) was significantly correlated with child fearfulness at school, and (*c*) father talkativeness combined with extreme levels of paternal affect displayed in the family room were significantly correlated with the child's distractible behavior at school.

Study 2: Analysis of Evaluative Consistency Across Communication Channels*

The second method of analyzing the family videotapes focused on the positive to negative evaluative dimension, comparing the evaluative qualities that were conveyed simultaneously in different channels of communication. Sample messages were analyzed with respect to the evaluative connotations rated separately for:

* A version of this study can be found in Bugental, Love, Kaswan, and April, 1971. © 1971 by the American Psychological Association and reprinted by permission.

1. The visual channel: facial expressions, gestures, etc., shown in the TV picture without sound.

2. The vocal channel: tone of voice as heard on videotapes without picture, with content removed by a band-pass filter.

3. The verbal channel: a script of what was actually said in the message.

The purpose of this analysis was to see whether there was greater evaluative inconsistency (e.g., an approving verbal statement accompanied by disapproving nonverbal behavior) in the communication of referred and nonreferred parents. This analysis is relevant to theoretical speculations, clinical observations, and research on the relation between conflicting parental communication and psychopathology in children. Much of the work in this area has been stimulated by the double-bind hypotheses of family interaction in schizophrenia (Bateson, Jackson, Haley, & Weakland, 1956; Weakland, 1961), but there has been increasing interest in the relation between inconsistent communication and more general psychological disturbances (e.g., Beakel & Mehrabian, 1969). Unfortunately, the double-bind hypothesis has received little empirical support (Schuham, 1968), and the evidence for conflict in parental messages to disturbed children is largely anecdotal. The only directly relevant empirical study we know of (Beakel & Mehrabian, 1969) focused on the relation between psychopathology in adolescence and congruence between the verbal and postural communication of evaluative meanings from parents to children. The study indicated parental messages to be more negative toward more disturbed, in comparison with less disturbed, adolescents. However, there was no relation demonstrated between psychopathology and verbal-postural incongruity in parents' messages to their children.

The same sample and the same judges were used in this analysis as in the previous one. Approximately 3 months intervened between the two sets of ratings. Reliability data is found in Appendix B, Table 13.

Videotapes of the 30 families were started at a random point and those parent-child messages were selected in which (a) the person speaking was visible, (b) only one person was speaking and the words could be clearly understood, and (c) the message had been rated independently by the two judges in the previous study as either positive or negative in total evaluative content. Whenever possible, one positive and one negative scene was obtained for each parent. Not all parents produced both positive and negative scenes but there were no R/NR differences in the average number of positive or negative scenes.

The following scenes are typical for length and type of message:

Encoder	Verbal Message
Nonreferred father	"I asked you to sit down. Now I won't ask you again."
Referred father	"How's your breathing today? Is your cold better today?"
Nonreferred mother	"Lookit, lookit that. Look at the other one. Those are not your socks."
Referred mother	"And then they'll take me and then you'll be left by yourself, Jimmy."

Independent ratings of the verbal, vocal, and visual channels were made for all scenes on the same 13 point evaluative scale used in the previous analysis. Ratings of the verbal content were obtained by having the judges rate typescripts of all scenes. For vocal ratings, the audio portion of the tape was played through a band-pass filter which rendered speech unintelligible. For visual ratings, the TV monitor was on but the sound was turned off.

Any channel input rated as positive (or negative) by at least four out of five judges was considered to be positive (or negative) in subsequent analyses. Any scene containing a consensually established positive message in one channel and a negative one in another was considered to represent a conflicting message. For example, if for a given scene (a) four out of five judges rated the picture as positive, (b) four out of five judges rated the script as negative, but (c) failed to agree (or gave neutral ratings) to the voice, the scene was categorized as demonstrating visual-verbal conflict. If, on the other hand, in the same situation, four out of five judges rated the voice as also negative, the scene would be categorized as demonstrating visual-vocal conflict as well as visual-verbal conflict.

REFERRED-NONREFERRED COMPARISONS

A higher proportion (67%) of referred parents produced conflicting messages than did nonreferred parents (30%), but the overall difference was not significant ($x^2 = 2.40$, $p < .20$, Appendix B, Table 14). A partitioning of groups by parent sex (see Appendix B, Table 15) reveals, however, that there is a significant difference between referred and nonreferred mothers (x^2, adjusted by Yates's correction for continuity, $= 4.32$, $p < .05$) but not between referred and nonreferred fathers (corrected $x^2 = 0.13$). *A much greater proportion of referred mothers (59%) produced conflicting messages than did nonreferred mothers (10%)*. This difference did not appear to be influenced by the presence or absence of a father in the home. "Conflicting" mothers were just as common in two-parent referred families (60%) as in father-absent referred families (57%). The conflicting messages produced by referred mothers included conflict between verbal content and facial expression, and between verbal content and tone of voice, but not between face and voice. There were no significant differences between groups in specific types of channel conflict manifested. The finding that the mothers of referred children give simultaneous conflicting evaluative messages in different communications channels is consistent with aspects of the double-bind hypothesis.

A common type of conflicting message produced by the mothers of disturbed children contained a critical or disapproving statement spoken in a positive voice. For example, one mother typically cooed all her criticisms, for example, "That's not n-i-c-e." If the mother was attempting to soften or deny the negative component in one channel by a positive component in another, her message was likely to be decided much more negatively by the child than she would anticipate. Some of our previous data (Bugental et al., 1970) suggest that young children resolve most conflicting messages by accepting the negative component and totally or partially discounting positive components, particularly in messages from women.

SOCIOECONOMIC LEVEL COMPARISONS

No SEL comparisons were made because of the small number of cases in the control group.

REFERRAL CATEGORY COMPARISONS

To examine how the referral problem of the child might be related to conflicting messages from referred mothers, the child's severity scores on the four categories were compared for those mothers who produced conflicting messages versus those who did not. There was a nonsignificant trend ($U = 20$, $p < .20$, two-tailed test) for the ratings on "aggressiveness" to be higher for the children of "conflicting" mothers than for the children of "nonconflicting" mothers. When comparisons were limited to boys, the difference between the two groups of mothers was statistically significant ($U = 6.5$, $p < .05$, two-tailed test). These aggressive children were described by their teachers as defiant, belligerent, and generally disruptive in the classroom and on the playground.

The conflicting communication patterns of their mothers may have the effect of arousing the negative feelings of the child (because of the negative evaluative component) while simultaneously inhibiting a direct negative response (because of the positive component). By giving a positive nonverbal message along with a verbal criticism, for example, the mother is saying, "I'm criticizing you but you shouldn't get angry with me because I'm really being nice." When children responded negatively to this type of disapproval, the mother often countered by telling the child he should not be resentful because she had his best interest at heart. The child was effectively constrained from responding with anger toward the mother but may have subsequently expressed his aggression in the "safer" school environment. This speculative interpretation seems related to the frustration-aggression hypothesis, since there was little evidence in our data of the child's modeling the mother.

No other relationships were found between referral category ratings and conflicting parental messages.

This method for studying contradictory messages seems to be a fruitful approach to an issue that has previously defied empirical analysis. When clinicians have reported contradictions in interpersonal messages or characteristics of interaction in families with disturbed children, it has been extremely difficult to specify empirically testable criteria for such messages (e.g., Mishler & Waxler, 1968, pp. 274–275). In large part this difficulty seems to result from the typical focus on linguistic patterns of contradiction which, because of problems like change in context and multiple levels of meaning, are virtually impossible to classify into a manageable number of nontrivial categories. Although the approach employed in the second study left out much of the richness of meaning that is possible when behavior is rated in context, it does refer to clinically meaningful aspects of contradiction in communication. In fact, recognition that divergent meanings are often conveyed in different channels is basic to the use of videotapes as a method for client-feedback and self-confrontation described in Chapters 7, 8, 9, and 10.

Integration of Findings from Videotape Analyses

Findings in the first of these two analyses reported emphasized the importance of the father's behavior, as have other measures in this study. Because our sample included a disproportionately large number of boys we cannot be certain to what extent our findings are accurate only for boys and to what extent they may hold for all children within this age range. Similar *trends,* however, were observed for families of girls as for the families of boys, and evidence from other research suggests that the father's behavior has a great deal of importance for both boys and girls (e.g., Hetherington, 1965).

Referred and nonreferred mothers were remarkably similar in the first study reported. In the second videotape study, however, subtle contradictions within communication channels, innuendos, nonverbal warnings, or encouragements, emerged as distinguishing indications of noncongruence, insincerity, or social role playing behavior in referred mothers. Thus these mothers teased, scolded indulgently, or made friendly verbal overtures that sounded like complaints. In general, they created a perplexing situation for the child in which it was unclear whether they were expressing approval or disapproval.

It is interesting to note that there were no differences or trends between referred and nonreferred mothers in global ratings on the evaluative dimension. The two groups were indistinguishable either in terms of average affect level or affective lability (extreme scores on the evaluative dimension). It may be that differential maternal behavior is better demonstrated at more subtle communication levels. Perhaps it may be necessary to focus on nonverbal communication or verbal-nonverbal interaction before differences between referred and nonreferred mothers can be observed, at least when maternal groups feel under pressure while being viewed and evaluated by professional psychologists.

An excerpt from the family interaction of the child with the highest severity scores in our sample (with a primary referral problem of aggressive behavior) may help to pull the reported differences together. The father was rated as negative, domineering, and evaluatively extreme. Additionally, the mother demonstrated high evaluative conflict between communication channels. The father's voice was consistently gruff and irritated and he slouched in his chair. The mother's voice was consistently indulgent and singsong while her posture and general appearance conveyed an impression of self-confidence. The three boys (aged 9, 12, and 15) were all oversized and muscular, typical "toughs" in speech and movement. (The family is focused on the fact that they are probably being observed and have been talking about the mirror and the microphone.)

Father: [to target boy, aged 9] The man from UNCLE [laughs].
Mother: Yeah.
Child: [to observation window] Hey, you can come in now.
Mother: Oh, Billy [condescending, indulgent voice].
Child: How come you have that mirror?
Father: [to child] What's the big dirt on your pants?
Mother: That's a stain . . . I can't get it out.
Child: How come they have these spies?
Mother: They're not spying . . . they're just observing.
Father: [to Sibling] I wish you'd brush your teeth . . . they're so yellow, honey.
[Sibling, aged 12, doesn't respond . . . turns away and draws mouth tight.]
Mother: [singing] You wonder where the yellow went . . . with Pepsodent [smiling] . . .

[Father reaches for and strokes Sibling's hand but boy pulls away.]
.
.
.

[Father becomes angry because of time wait.]

Child [repeats over and over in singsong voice]: The computers are running down.
.
.
.
.
.
.
.
.
.
.

Mother: I think it is very interesting don't you? [smiles]

Father: If I don't get to bed until 11:00 . . . I just can't stand it . . . and then go to work tomorrow . . . I don't feel too good anyway.

Mother: Oh, Harvey [same condescending voice as used with child].

[Father turns away.]

Mother: You're always such a humbug.

Father: [to child] Do you think they are observing at you, Billy?

[Boy talks about canned juice in room.]

Child: It's probably doped.

Mother: Oh, Billy, Billy, Billy.

Father: Maybe they've got something in there to make you goofy or something.

Mother: So you want to talk.

Father: Gee that's terrible.
         Maybe it's a trick . . . huh, Billy?

[Boy shrugs but sits and looks at father intently.]

Father: They're all watching now . . . hey, wouldn't it be a good show . . . you're on Candid Camera.

[Boy looks at microphone and shoots it with finger.]

Child: I'll pull out my pistol.

Father: I wish you had your bongo and your little tape recorder so you could give them a little . . .

The observed family interaction patterns that distinguished between referred and nonreferred families also differentiated among referral categories, that is, children who had different presenting problems came from families with different patterns of communication. Children who were aggressive in school were likely to have fathers who were rated as directive and interpersonally negative in the family room and mothers who produced evaluatively conflicting messages, as in the above example. These two findings support and amplify previous observations that the parents of aggressive children are rejecting and inconsistent (McCord, et al., 1961; Bandura & Walters, 1959). The inconsistency of the mother and the negativity of the father in families of aggressive children should not be viewed as independent occurrences. These two sets of parental behaviors were found to be significantly related to each other, and the following interrelations appear:

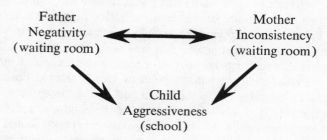

The parents' behavior may have a causal relationship to the child's behavior in school, but it is unclear whether the mother is responding to the father or the father is responding to the mother, or both. Further analysis of sequences of behavior will be required before the interaction of the two parental behaviors can be fully understood.

Apparently, family interaction patterns demonstrated in 5 minutes of free interaction reflect sufficient variability to identify not only referred and nonreferred families, but also, to some extent, different referral categories for the child. The initial differences are maintained over longer periods as well. This is doubly important to note since few R/NR differences were found in the children's own behavior on the tapes. Results from other instruments in this study indicate that referred and nonreferred families *do* see differences in the children's behavior at home. It seems probable that the clinic setting may have had a sufficiently restraining effect on the children's behavior to obviate R/NR differences. Presumably, the behavior of the parents was also more constrained at the clinic than at home so that the observed R/NR differences may be an underestimate of typical differences in the behavior of these groups (e.g., Lennard & Bernstein, 1969).

CHAPTER 5

The Child at School

The child's behavior in the school setting was studied through measures that paralleled two of the family instruments: adjective ratings and behavior inventories. Teachers' perceptions of the child at school were sampled through adjective scales and a questionaire that was an abbreviated parallel to the Parent Behavior Inventory. To provide a second impression of the child at school (from other than a teacher's point of view), trained observers also rated the child's behavior in the classroom and on the playground, using the standard adjectives. The adults' perceptions of the children in terms of each instrument are presented in the usual comparisons between R and NR children, children at different SELs, and in the four referral categories.

TEACHER ADJECTIVE RATINGS

Teachers' ratings were completed during an interview between the teacher and a project worker scheduled as soon as a child had been identified for participation in the project. Like other raters, the teacher was first given the Semantic Differential for the individual adjectives. She* then rated "the average child in my class," "the target child" (by name), and her expectations as to how this child would rate her. All ratings used the standard 9 point "never-always" scale and the denotative definitions of the adjectives. In the same session the teacher had an opportunity to give additional information about the child and to ask questions about her own participation in the study. Three project workers conducted all teacher interviews and gave the same basic information and orientation to all teachers. Means and analyses of all teacher ratings are given in Appendix B, Tables 16, 17, and 18. Additional details regarding the teacher scales are presented in Appendix A, pp. 247–248.

* Though there were a few male teachers involved, our teacher group consisted primarily of women.

Referred—Nonreferred Comparisons

Differences between teacher ratings of the R and NR children were highly significant ($p < .01$) on both factors, with the referred children always receiving the less favorable rating: higher scores for Negative Social Impact, lower scores for positive social assets. Since the teachers had been intimately involved in the identification of all children, this was the expected finding. Ratings made of "the average child in my classroom" showed that the teachers apparently had a highly consistent concept of the "average" pupil: they used the middle of the scale on all concepts. Whether teachers had only a referred child in their classrooms (as was the case for two-thirds of them) or had one referred and one control child in their classes (for each of whom they made separate ratings at different times), there were no significant differences in ratings of the "average" child. This finding provides some evidence that there were no generalized special expectations, or biased sensitivities with respect to children's behavior, that characterized either teacher group. (At least none were sufficiently generalized to be reflected in these adjective ratings.)

Socioeconomic Level Comparisons

Teachers gave relatively high ratings to both groups of Lo SEL children, referred and nonreferred, for socially negative characteristics. (The SEL effect was significant at $p < .05$.) Additional material is noted later which reflects teachers' perceptions of undesirable characteristics of Lo SEL children in their behavior inventories, as well as in their adjective ratings. Although Lo SEL children were frequently referred for problems of aggression (see Chapter 2), this category was also frequent for referred Hi SEL children. Still, teachers tended to perceive both Mid and Hi SEL children as having significantly less negative impact than Lo SEL pupils.

For the Positive Impact ratings, there were no significant differences in teachers' views of children at different socioeconomic levels. Teachers had apparently discriminated "defects" in behavior at different SELs more generally than they differentiated levels of adaptive, effective functioning. This may have occurred because they knew they were participating in a clinical study in which referred children would receive psychological treatment: they may have adopted a "symptom" orientation on this basis. Furthermore the identification criterion of the control children (that they not manifest any major behavior or emotional difficulty) would tend to evoke this set. But the basic R/NR comparisons, as described in the preceding discussion, were highly significant on *both* factors. So something related to socioeconomic variables seemed to cloud the teachers' differentiation of children's adaptive functioning.

Referral Category Comparisons

For the referred children, teachers had filled out detailed descriptions of each child's difficulties at the time of referral. Table 1 shows the mean adjective ratings on the two factors for children classified on the basis of their predominant referral category.

Table 1.   Mean Adjective Ratings on Two Factors for Children Classified in their Predominant Referral Categories

Social Impact of Child's Behavior	Ag	Hy	SW	AC
Negative	6.14	6.28	4.06	4.99
Positive	4.03	3.55	3.36	3.34

Mean ratings for negativity were different between referral groups at $p < .01$, Appendix B, Table 17. There were low scores for socially withdrawn children but high scores for hyperactive and aggressive children, as is predictable from the definition of these categories. Differences between groups on the positive factor were not significant, though the means suggest that aggressive children tended to be seen in more positive (friendly, active, controlling, not bored) terms than other referred children. Teachers' ratings again proved to be more discriminating for symptomatic behaviors (negative factor) than for socially desirable characteristics of children's school behavior.

An index of the degree of perceived deviance of the various disturbances from usual or expected school behavior was studied by comparing teacher ratings of the referred children with her ratings of "average" children. Predictably the "average" child was seen as less negative and more positive in his social behavior than the problem groups. *Hyperactive and aggressive behaviors were most negatively deviant, whereas attention control problems were quite close to the norm on this factor, with socially withdrawn children appearing less negative than the "average" child.* Differences in positive characteristics were less clear. Hyperactive and socially withdrawn children were seen as slightly less positive, in comparison to the average, than aggressive and distractible children.

Teacher's Expectations of How the Child Will Rate Her

In specifying her expectations as to how the individual child would rate her, the teacher clearly indicated that the referred child would perceive her in significantly more negative terms than would the nonreferred. For the social negativity factor, the difference (R > NR) was significant at $p < .05$. For the child's ratings of her friendliness, activity, etc., she expected a much clearer difference between groups: R < NR at $p < .001$. The fact that the teacher had referred the disturbed child to outsiders indicated that her own efforts to help had been at least partly unsuccessful. In many cases discomfort between child and teacher had built up to such levels that the teacher would naturally expect the child to see her as angry and impatient on the one hand and not very friendly or involved on the other. In comparison to the child's actual ratings of her, however, the teacher's sensitivity far exceeded the child's reaction. The mean ratings of their teachers made by referred children were more favorable than those made by control children, but these R/NR differences were not statistically significant ($p < .20$ for the negative, $p < .10$ for the positive factor, Appendix B, Table 19). This, in conjunction with their similarly positive ratings of their parents on the FARS, indicates that even the troubled children in this age range remain relatively favorable in their expressed evaluation of the significant adults in their lives. We have no data as to whether any "safety versus sincerity" factor might be represented in these ratings.

There were no statistically significant differences in SEL or referral category analyses of teachers' expectations of pupils' ratings.

Summary of Teacher Adjective Ratings

Teachers' use of the adjective scales differentiated referred and nonreferred groups in expected directions on both positive and negative attributes of interpersonal activity. In their predictions of how they would be rated, teachers anticipated much more unfavorable ratings from referred than from nonreferred children. Their expectations of negative evaluation from the troubled children proved to be greater than the dissatisfaction these youngsters actually expressed in their teacher ratings.

Teachers rated Lo SEL children (R and NR) higher on negativity than either Mid or Hi SELs. Teachers in Lo SEL schools discriminated R/NR differences on problem behaviors (Negative Social Impact) for the children but reflected no difference between referred and nonreferred groups on Positive Social Impact. A somewhat negative perception of Lo SEL children seems generally reflected in the teacher ratings.

TEACHER BEHAVIOR INVENTORY

Since teachers could give relatively little time to project measures, a brief form of the Parent Behavior Inventory was developed for teacher use. Whenever content could be translated appropriately from the family to the school context, PBI items covering the child's behavior (adaptive as well as symptomatic) were transferred to the teacher inventory. In addition, items specific to the school situation were added to delineate the quality and circumstances of his activity in the classroom, on the playground, in relation to the teacher, and in relation to his peers.

Unfortunately, school administrators had required that teacher behavior not be a direct focus of our work; TBI items were therefore limited to child behavior. The Teacher Inventory is reproduced in Appendix B, Table 20; a discussion of the statistical procedures utilized is contained in Appendix A, p. 248.

Referred—Nonreferred Comparisons

The results are summarized in Table 2, which is constructed like the Parent Behavior Inventory tables. Nine of the 14 factors in this table show significant differences between the referred and the nonreferred groups. Since the referral of the children was initiated by school personnel, always including the teacher, these differences are to be expected and indicate, more specifically than the referral category labels, the behaviors that led up to referral. As in the Parent Behavior Inventory, *referred children, as compared to the nonreferred group, were rated as less interpersonally effective (factor 2), less affiliative (14), more immature (8), insecure (9), and sensitive to ridicule and rejection (4). They were much more often involved in interpersonal conflict, on both verbal and physical levels, and involving both peers and teachers (1). Their discontents were expressed over a broad range of verbal complaints and antisocial behaviors, including stealing and breaking objects (10). Whereas the activity patterns of control children were constructive and represented autonomous task organization (13), referred children's high level of activity reflected anxious, nervous mannerisms (5).*

Teachers thus cataloged major differences between the two child groups which centered on developmental levels and on the amount and quality of interpersonal behavior. They reported more differences in children's relationships with peers than variations in the quality of their pupils' interactions with themselves.

The *evaluative* differences in the teachers' Behavior Inventories consistently favored the control children, in the expected direction in all comparisons. The indices of children's *activity* patterns emphasized the organized, self-directed quality of nonreferred children who operated at moderate, consistent levels. This is in contrast to referred children's activity styles which took two patterns: a set of highly active, nervous, aggressive behaviors on the one hand, and a group of low active, anxious, insecure behaviors on the other. No direct *power* relationships are spelled out thus far, but some implications will be inferred in the context of additional data.

Socioeconomic Level Comparisons

There were no significant main SEL effects in analyses of variance of Teacher Behavior Inventory factors. When SEL differences in referred families were compared with the pattern of SEL differences within the control group, however, a significant interaction ($p < .05$) between a child's SEL and his membership in either the referred or nonreferred group appeared for the combined mean of the four factors dealing with his interpersonal adaptiveness (2, 11, 12, 14). The general pattern is that among referred children, those in Hi SEL schools are more socially handicapped than are youngsters from Lo SEL backgrounds. For control children the opposite is true: the higher the child's SEL, the more favorable the picture gained of his interpersonal competence in the school setting. The four factors involved the child's interpersonal effectiveness, happiness, responsiveness to rewards, and affiliation tendencies.

The number of cases in these subgroups is quite small when the nonreferred cases are separated into SEL groups, and there was no significant main effect, but the interaction obtained seems consistent and strong enough over the different factors to suggest that the finding is not accidental. Also, this finding parallels results obtained in the teacher adjective ratings where Lo SEL referred children were seen to have more Positive Social Impact than Hi SEL referred children. The reverse trend was obtained for nonreferred children. These results suggest some recognition by the teacher that the acting out, aggressive behavior which they ascribe to Lo SEL children is not a uniform pattern of uncontrolled hostility. Just as Lo SEL referred parents recognized that, in spite of their children's recalcitrance in the family, they were socially effective outside the home (Parent Behavior Inventory), so the teacher seemed to indicate that Lo SEL children are disturbing to her in the classroom, but may be highly effective with their peers.

Referral Category Comparisons

Teachers made some differential evaluations of children's negativity that were associated with their predominant problems. Differences between referral category were also related to children's activity patterns in terms of their potential disruption of the learning situation, since children who were socially withdrawn were rated as much less negative than those who were aggressive and hyperactive.

Table 2. Summary of Significant Comparison—Teacher Behavior Inventory

Factor No.	Content			Referral Category			
		R (N=59)	NR (N=26)	Ag (N=12)	Hy (N=10)	SW (N=11)	AC (N=26)
	Interpersonal adaptiveness						
2	Interpersonal effectiveness: leader, liked, effective, dependable	<*					<*Ag
14	Peer affiliation: helpful, sociable, compliant, team member	<*			<*Ag		
11	Responsiveness to rewards: likes time with teacher, presents, praise	<*		>*SW			
12	Happiness: shown by laughing, whistling, excitement, etc.						
	Interpersonal problems						
8	Immaturity: plays with younger children, refuses direction, poor hand coordination	>*					
9	Insecurity: shows anger and worry by crying; upset when paid no attention	>**					
3	Dependency: seeks reassurance, affection from teacher						

4　Oversensitivity: upset by interpersonal rejection, being laughed at, criticism　>*　　　　>*SW　　>*SW　　<*Ag

Hostility

1　Interpersonal conflict: verbally and physically attacked by peers; attacks peers, teacher　>**

10　Destructiveness: breaks things, steals, complains, whines　>*

Control and reaction to control

7　Manipulative: flatters, bribes to gain teacher, peer acceptance

6　Resistance to direction: performs as asked after threats, bribery

Motor Behavior

13　Dexterity, self-sufficiency: good with hands, happy working alone　<*

5　Nervous activity: noisy, active, bites nails, upset when alone　>**　　>*SW　　>*AC　　<*Hy　　<*Ag

*t=p < .05.
**t=p < .01.

123

Referral category differences were obtained on four factors. All comparisons were at the $p < .05$ significance level.

Interpersonal Conflict: is verbally and physically attacked by peers; attacks peers, teacher.
Ag > SW; Hy > SW
Ag > AC
Aggressive and hyperactive children are involved in more interpersonal conflict than are socially withdrawn children. Aggressive children exceed distractible children in becoming embroiled in conflict.

Nervous Activity: is noisy, active, bites nails, is upset when alone.
Ag > AC; Hy > AC
Ag > SW
Aggressive and hyperactive children engage in much more nervous activity than do inhibited and distractible children.

Interpersonal Effectiveness: is a leader, is liked, is effective, dependable.
Ag > Hy
Ag > SW
Aggressive children are seen as more interpersonally effective, especially with peers, than are hyperactive or socially withdrawn children.

Peer Affiliation: is helpful, sociable, a compliant team member.
Ag > SW
Aggressive children turn to peers more than do socially inhibited children.

These results seem self-evident and demonstrate the consistency of the teachers' observations of children's behavior at school. They also reflect the attention the teacher pays to the children's activity patterns and to the amount and type of interpersonal relations children maintain with their peers.

The results point up basic similarities in the teacher's description of aggressive and hyperactive children on the one hand, and socially withdrawn and distractible children on the other. Aggressive and hyperactive children are active, reach out to others, and have significant impact on them. When this effect is negative, it takes the form of either conflict with teacher and peers, or nervous, unproductive activity. The socially withdrawn or distractible children, on the other hand, avoid interpersonal contact, whether friendly or unfriendly, and seem to be in a state of internal discomfort that inhibits and disorganizes their behavior.

With respect to the three basic behavioral dimensions (activity, directing, and evaluating components), the interpersonally oriented aggressive and hyperactive children vary across extremes of positive and negative interactions.

Their activity levels are quite high and whether directed toward constructive goals or toward reduction of high tension levels, they have high interpersonal impact. The other children evoke intermediate evaluative judgments and are low in their activity levels as well as in their tolerance for interpersonal involvements. They are diffident and ineffective in interactions with their peers, and dependent and compliant with adults. They thus generally adopt a low power position in their interpersonal stance.

SCHOOL OBSERVERS' ADJECTIVE RATINGS

By prearrangement with teachers and administrators in all schools, pairs of project observers rated children's behavior in the school setting without the observed child's knowledge and before referred or nonreferred children had any awareness of the project. These observations were intended to provide information about the children's behavior at school from the viewpoint of someone other than school personnel. Since they would be repeated at later intervals, they were also intended to be a major outcome criterion in comparing behavioral changes associated with the three types of treatment that would be provided for the referred children in the clinic.

The paid raters were parent-aged women, most of whom had children of elementary-school age. They were largely without background in the mental health field, as we were seeking naive observers who would hopefully respond to the behavior they saw, and make a minimum of inferences about their observations. The only information given them was that this was a study of the behavior of school children. They were asked explicitly not to inquire or speculate about the purpose of their ratings, in order to minimize the development of bias. A pool of from five to eight raters was available for these ratings.

They were trained in the school situation, initially rating 8–10 nonsample children and comparing their ratings with concurrent ratings made by senior project personnel. They used the regular 10-adjective rating scale, always with reference to the standard denotative definitions. Training focused their attention on the children's overt behaviors. Their ratings were checked weekly for the first month, then about every 2 weeks, by comparing their ratings with those of the project school liasion worker on one or two nonsample children.

At any one rating session, two raters observed the same two children without knowledge of their classification.* One was a referred child, the oth-

---

* In the early phase of first year observations, there were some cases in which one rater was not "blind." Procedures were altered and a Year I by Year II analysis indicates that there was no significant difference between the two years' ratings.

er either a nonreferred or randomly selected child. This last group of children, the "randoms," were included both to provide a wider base for the observers' ratings and to reduce the likelihood of their identification of R/NR group differences in the children. The project liaison workers arranged in advance for the teacher's unobtrusive designation of the children to be rated in each session.

Ratings were made in three contexts: *in the classroom*, the observers rated the child *in relation to peers and, separately, to the teacher*. The total period of classroom observation lasted from 30 to 50 minutes. Immediately after each observation period, the raters completed their ratings independently of each other. In the third context the school observers rated the child's *behavior in relation to peers on the playground*. To make these ratings, the observers followed the class onto the playground during a recess, remaining close enough to be able to watch the identified children's interactions, but staying far enough away so as not to indicate who was being observed. Verbal behavior often could not be assessed in these interactions, so that "clear" was not rated and not included in the analyses.

In addition to adjective ratings, classroom observation included 5 point scale ratings ("not at all" to "very much") of *(a)* task involvement—how much of the time and how exclusively the child paid attention to the teacher or carried out classroom assignments; *(b)* social play—amount of time and degree to which child was involved with other children apart from classroom assignments, *(c)* divergence—amount of time and degree to which the child was engaged in self-oriented activity, like staring into space, fantasy play, or self-stimulation in the classroom; *(d)* amount of time the child participated in assigned games on the playground; and *(e)* extent to which the child played alone, wandered around by himself, sat alone, or avoided the playground.

Interrater agreement was above .70 in more than three-quarters of the ratings. Details of the techniques and results for assessing reliability of school observers' ratings are found in Appendix A, pp. 248–249 along with the statistical treatments and results upon which this discussion is based.

Analyses of school observers' ratings of the children followed the usual pattern. Since they rated each child three times, in three different contexts, and during 2 years of data collection, there is a large number of comparisons. Information on those most directly relevant to parent and teacher ratings are found in Appendix B, Tables 21 and 22.

Referred—Nonreferred Comparisons

Overall differences in adjective ratings were analyzed separately for each factor with a Group (R, NR) Year (1st, 2nd) Context (child-teacher, child-peers, child-playground) analysis of variance. *On the Negative Social Impact factor, school observers identified the referred children as significantly higher than the control children* (R > NR, *p* < .001), though differences were always greater for playground than classroom ratings. The original identification of the referred children was apparently based upon children's behaviors that would seem troubled to nonprofessional women. They thus did not seem due to bias on the part of school personnel.

Just as teachers had made more R/NR discriminations of children's negative impact than of their positive adaptive qualities, so the school observers failed to identify significant differences between the child groups in terms of differential social effectiveness in any of the three rating situations. As with teachers, school observers knew nothing of the purpose or goals of the study. However, they obtained their daily school assignments from project staff in the Psychology Clinic, and may have assumed a "clinical" slant as a consequence. In any case, *a persistent, pervasive focus on children's negative qualities seems an easily evoked adult orientation.* In family ratings it may be recalled that differentiations were made of both positive and negative qualities, but children were always perceived more negatively than adults. There is more than a hint in these findings that children are born "bad" and that the path toward social "goodness" is a slow and laborious one, watched over with somewhat jaundiced adult eyes. It should be recalled here that the nonreferred parents' openly expressed high regard and respect for their child's personal and interpersonal attributes was a major characteristic differentiating them from referred parents. This point is epitomized in the control father's enjoyment of active involvement with his child.

In addition to the adjective ratings, school observers made global ratings of each child's task orientation in class, his divergence from group activities (daydreaming, playing alone, etc.) and his disruptive behavior in classroom and playground. Along such behavioral dimensions, observers rated referred and nonreferred children as significantly different (*p* < .05) in the expected direction: *the control children were more task oriented, less divergent in the class, and less disruptive on the playground than the referred children.* Thus there is agreement between all adults (observers, teachers, and parents) in their evaluations of R and NR children on these dimensions. However, the school observers did not identify significant differences in the amount of task-disruptive social play engaged in by the two groups in the classroom.

Socioeconomic Level Comparisons

There were no significant SEL differences found in the observers' ratings. It may be that this result is a consequence of the instructions given them to

128   The Child at School

rate observed behavior, without inference insofar as possible. Compliance with these instructions would mean that their comparative framework for any rating would be limited to other children in the immediate situation. These would always be other children at the same SEL, as was described in Chapter 2. This restriction might decrease comparison with children from different social and cultural backgrounds. In any case the *results emphasize the similarity of children's school behaviors across SEL at this age range and suggest that our school observers made ratings free of social class expectations or bias.*

Referral Category Comparisons

The school raters' observations were the planned means for checking on the validity of the referral categorizations (which were based on teachers' reports of the referred childrens' school behaviors). Though teachers presumably made their judgments over a considerable period of time, we assumed that if the problems were indeed serious and chronic, they should be observable even during the brief periods available to our raters. But the analyses of observer ratings do not substantiate this expectation at statistically significant levels. Since referral statements from the teachers had clearly emphasized the situational basis of many concerns about the child (emphasis on attention control problems, for instance), instructional needs may have resulted in descriptions of the referred children that would not be immediately shared by adults who did not have a "teaching" responsibility or orientation. Nevertheless, it is surprising that basic behavioral differences were not salient for the raters. Their presence as outside observers may have had some damping effect on the children's deviant behavior, even though they did not know they were being specially observed; however, this is conjectural.

Though the overall referral category effects were not statistically significant, the pattern of means for Negative Social Impact repeats the previously defined parallel between aggressive and hyperactive children vis-à-vis the socially withdrawn and distractible youngsters (Appendix B, Table 22). Teachers' ratings and responses had reflected these two sets of alignments within the four referral categories. School observers further indicated that in a constrained situation determined by adult-child relations (i.e., in the classroom) the hyperactive and aggressive groups vary together and in opposite directions from the withdrawn and distractible children. In the classroom the interpersonally oriented children were more likely to behave in rude, angry, phony, impatient ways, as compared to the quieter, less socially involved groups, and thus to receive unfavorable ratings. On the playground, however, where peer relationships were dominant, the interpersonally oriented children displayed their social assets effectively and received more favorable evaluations from school observers. No marked differences appeared in the classroom versus playground behavior of the interpersonally avoidant children. Though this pattern seems consistent and is substantiated by the teacher data, it should be remembered that in these observers' ratings the comparisons did not achieve statistical significance.

In summary, there is general accord in the picture of overall R/NR differences, as recorded by teachers and school observers. Teachers, unlike the observers, reflected a more negative perception of Lo SEL children than those of Mid or Hi SELs; but teachers also judged Lo SEL referred children to have higher positive impact than Hi SEL referred pupils. Both groups of adult female raters differentiated the aggressive and hyperactive children's patterns from those of the socially inhibited and distractible children. Finally, both rater groups made more discriminations in negative than positive aspects of children's functioning. This is in contrast to family measures where the FARS especially reflected more R/NR differences in positive as compared to negative ratings.

CHAPTER 6

Integration of Family and School Findings

This chapter draws together major findings of our four assessment techniques with respect to pretreatment characteristics of (1) individual family members, (2) parental patterns, and (3) the child in the family and at school, considering both similarities and differences in the type of information gained from our various measures. Family Adjective Rating Scales and Parent Behavior Inventories are verbal assessments of the interpersonal regard and behavior of family members in daily life. The Family Communication Task is a recorded sample of interchanges between family members while they are engaged in an impersonal, cognitive, usually highly interesting verbal task. The fourth source of data, videotapes, shows the total family interacting in an observed setting which usually induces some degree of tension or constraint in everyone. Within the framework of the different situations represented by the four techniques, behavior in referred and nonreferred families is described in its activity, directing, and evaluation connotations.

PATTERNS OF PARENTAL BEHAVIOR

Referred—Nonreferred Differences

FATHERS

Referred and nonreferred fathers were found to differ consistently in all four sets of data and on each of the three interpersonal dimensions.

Nonreferred fathers were characterized by high levels of positive interaction with both their wives and children in familial descriptions of daily life patterns (FARS and PBI). In a problem-solving situation in the clinic (the communication task) they demonstrated this activity directly. Easy leadership was manifested in their instrumental behavior as the control fathers "took over," asked questions, and initiated effective communication. In the circumstance of being observed and recorded in the family room, their activity level decreased to lower levels of poise or detachment. They appeared relatively calm and confident, for themselves and their families. They rarely showed extremes of feeling and exerted few efforts to influence or control the children, leaving the operational management of seating arrangements, coat removal, preparation of snacks, etc., up to the mothers. They often indicated some self-consciousness with a wry, humorous recognition of a realistic sense of constraint, and sometimes were obviously uncomfortable; but observation did not seem to mobilize them to either defensive or aggressive maneuvers. They did not demonstrate the ingratiation, anxiety, or anger conveyed by referred fathers' expressive extremes in the family room.

Nonreferred fathers demonstrated their power with low levels of *effort* but high levels of *effect* in the father-child relationship in all situations. In general, these fathers received highest evaluation for their social effectiveness from their children (adjective ratings), and they in turn described their youngsters as highly responsive to their approval or disapproval (Parent Behavior Inventory). The children respected and sought paternal judgments (Behavior Inventory), and followed their effective lead in the communication task. In the videotaped interaction these fathers manifested little effort to exert power. Even so, for nonreferred fathers there was a positive correlation between talkativeness and directiveness: when they did speak, their messages were seen as having substantial directive qualities (videotape ratings). The consistency of this pattern across all measures implies a very stable, well-established, close, and mutually satisfying father-child relationship, with clearly defined paternal authority and responsibility.

In relationship to their wives, control fathers seemed to rely on mutual adaptation between the pair rather than efforts at interpersonal influence or dominance (PBI). Here mutual respect and confidence that each would do fairly and well by himself and by the other seemed in evidence (FARS). The relative degree of interpersonal trust and consideration reported on verbal measures was exemplified in parental actions in both the communication task and videotaped interactions, with each parent deferring to the other in role-appropriate areas.

Despite the evident differences that would attend different purposes in bringing their families to the clinic (nonreferred fathers were doing something *for* the observing clinicians; referred fathers presumably hoped the clinicians would do something for or about their children), the marked differences between these paternal roles and patterns are noteworthy.

The basically negative quality of the referred father's feeling tone in life situations was reported in their adjective ratings (given and received) and in the anxious complaints and critical descriptions they provided of their wives and children in the behavior inventory. In their daily lives, the referred fathers were described as spending little time in shared activities with their families (PBI) and their inventory responses indicated that they felt that they and their children did not know or understand each other well.

Their inventories also specified their use of a variety of techniques in efforts to influence others' behavior. These included both directly active demands and passive appeals to sympathy or guilt. We have no direct evidence of their effectiveness in this regard, but the reported (PBI) lack of mutual understanding, high marital conflict, and absence of joint social activity, together with the ineffectual behavior observed in the clinic, all indicate that these fathers did not achieve mutually satisfactory relationships within their families. Indeed both the mothers and the children rated and described them in relatively negative terms.

Thus referred fathers seemed to receive little expression of admiration or respect from the rest of their families. In comparison with their wives, especially, they were viewed by all members of the family as operating at low levels of interpersonal effectiveness, a characteristic which would seem an essential ingredient of successful instrumental functioning for interactions both within and outside the family. That they desired to appear interpersonally competent was evident in their expectations of high adjective ratings from their wives on this score. It was also demonstrated in their reports of sporadic assumptions of high power positions with both wives and children (PBI). When presented with the instrumental-cognitive situation of the communication task in the clinic, however, they did not display the activity or leadership shown by nonreferred fathers. In this lack of initiative, they gave a firsthand demonstration of ineffectualness in an area in which paternal leadership is often expected (problem-solving behavior). Similarly, under the pressure of interacting with their family while being observed, they further departed from the control fathers' confident role, exhibiting instead the behavior characteristic of mothers: the anxious, intrusive, directing behaviors often related to family management and emotional-expressive concerns. Our analyses, so far, do not indicate the basis for this behavior. Some fathers seemed to feel unable to be effective in their own right and so sought to imitate and compete with their wives. In other instances, they appeared to be responding to expectations held, and sometimes explicitly verbalized, by their wives: that they *should* be ready and able to take over and manage any situation on cue from their wives. There often seemed simultaneous implications in messages from these wives that their husbands should, but wouldn't, be able to carry out their paternal responsibilities satisfactorily.

Referred fathers expressed much anxiety and frustration with their famili-al position. In a few instances, they exploded into shouts and threats of physical attack in efforts to rebut their wives and/or children. Such out-bursts were sometimes intense enough to produce fear and temporary com-pliance within the family. Even then, though, their control was momentary and was obtained at the evident cost of further reduction in positive regard or respect: they were visibly further excluded by all family members thereafter.

Thus referred fathers' control attempts seemed related to the low levels of respect for their interpersonal competence that were expressed by their wives and children. These men appeared to seek high positive status in the family. Lacking this, demonstrably, they exerted pressure in a wide range of efforts to gain it. But they were unable to make their efforts effective. If they used force, they lost positive regard. If they complained, they were usually ignored. If they were supplicant, they were derided or disdained. Both the wives and children directly or indirectly repudiated their control attempts and sought to establish a position of competence or consequence for themselves. The resulting struggles for control depict a relatively struc-tureless, limitless environment for the child.

MOTHERS

Nonreferred mothers were obviously different from referred mothers on both sets of verbal reports and on the Family Communication Task. Differences in the family room behavior of the two maternal groups were not immediately evident, showing up only in detailed analyses of incongruity between their verbal and nonverbal behavior. On no instruments were the differences between mothers as pronounced as those between father groups. This holds especially for their descriptions of their own behavior with the child on their Behavior Inventories.

In terms of verbal reports of their daily behavior, NR mothers appeared to adopt a less active and directive role within the family than did R moth-ers. The latter expressed more demands on husbands and children, whether overtly or indirectly (PBI). They described themselves as more active with their children than did the NR mothers on the one hand, or their own hus-bands on the other (PBI). These behavioral descriptions were matched by the adjective ratings R mothers received: while the control mothers were rated at lower levels of Positive Social Impact by themselves and their chil-dren, the R mothers were given highest ratings on this score by both hus-bands and children. However, they did not themselves subscribe to this high evaluation of their interpersonal impact; instead they gave themselves a low-er rating, one which matched (was not significantly different from) the self-rating of the control mothers. Since they did not seem to see themselves as high in such terms as *active, friendly, controlling,* and *not bored,* there seems a possibility that the R mothers behaved in a more active and controlling style than they recognized.

On the evaluative dimension, the control mothers expressed and received more positive attributions than did referreds (ratings on Negative Social Impact and the PBI responses of both parents). However, no group difference for positive or negative behavior was revealed in judges' ratings of maternal behavior in the videotapes. This discontinuity is discussed below.

The NR mother verbally attributed generalized competence to her husband (FARS, PBI) and in the communication task in the clinic she deferred to his leadership role in this instrumental activity. In the same situations the referred mother ceded nothing to her spouse. She attributed low levels of interpersonal competence to him (FARS), and described a relatively dominant role for herself in relationship to him (PBI). In the family task she did not wait for her husband to take the lead. Instead, both parents talked, interrupting each other frequently in their attempts to seek information from the child. As a consequence the R mother appeared to be either competing with her husband for leadership in what might be considered a paternal function, or evidencing her expressed lack of trust in his ability to perform adequately. If it were the latter, she stepped in to make up in advance for his anticipated deficiencies.

In the videotaped interactions, both groups of mothers seemed highly responsive to having their family observed by psychologists and both behaved in highly controlling styles, especially in relationship to the children, grooming, criticizing, and managing them in numerous ways. As indicated, the NR father accepted this behavior on the wife's part as her appropriate responsibility, and left the field to her. The R father, however, reacted in comparable, and therefore apparently competitive, ways. Just as the R wife appeared to compete in instrumental functions (FARS, PBI, and leadership in the communication task), so the R father appeared to attempt to take over child management and expressive functions in the family room. *These two instances seem to represent role competition or role reversal, the latter a pattern of parental behavior that has been widely discussed but has seldom been clearly demonstrated* (e.g., Caputo, 1963). It is alternatively possible, however, that R mothers somehow involved their husbands in a type of indirect control, encouraging them to express some of the wives' own negativity (on which they considered themselves low). Project workers often felt that R fathers were seeking to do their wives' bidding, or to gain their acceptance or approval in their efforts to direct and control the child. In many instances it seemed that the mothers gave fathers the responsibility for managing the children when difficulties arose, while somehow withholding the authority that would permit them to be successful. Most referred mothers did not appear to back up or support paternal efforts at discipline or control.

The expressive extremes conveyed by both groups of mothers and by the referred fathers in the family room suggest that a relatively high level of affect was experienced by these three groups while being observed. Highly positive and approving, as well as highly negative and disapproving, behaviors were exhibited. Since positive expressions by referred parents appeared only in this public situation, the possibility is raised that these highly approving behaviors were related to being observed. (An anecdotal note contributes to this possibility: project staff viewing the videotapes quickly learned that sudden smiles on parents'—especially mothers'—faces often indicated that a project member had entered the family room at that point.) This observation supports others that imply a tendency for people to produce socially desirable responses to, or for, the presumed observers.

It is conjectured that all mothers and the R fathers may have responded to observation as a challenge to demonstrate their success in "handling" family life and child behavior in particular. In this sense it seemed a threat to self-regard and they became highly active, and affective, in the face of this threat. Such a possible tendency to seek external validation of their parental and marital effectiveness suggests a lack of inner satisfaction and security with respect to their familial roles. The implied pattern is that when there has been positive, effective activity in outside life, there is less need to demonstrate activity in the test case of being observed. When conflict, ineffectualness, and dissatisfaction had been characteristic of familial transactions, high levels of activity appeared in the observed situation, seemingly representing competing parental claims to being approving, competent, and in control. Under these circumstances, the expected role differentiations of the R parents (which often seemed blurred, even in verbal reports) failed to materialize and mutual role reversals appeared, resulting in competition and conflict for parents and inconsistency and loss of structure for children.

The high activity manifested by control mothers in the family room (in distinction to the more passive role described as their daily patterns) may indicate the well-known difficulty mothers experience in giving up controlling behavior as children grow up. It is surmised that residual directive tendencies may be relatively latent in life situations but that these may reemerge, even for generally effective mothers, under the stress of professional observation and evaluation.

We noted earlier that referred mothers used largely overt, direct demands in their attempts to influence their husbands but that they used both high and low power appeals with their children (PBI). It might be surmised on this basis that the R mothers were in a more secure power status in relation to their husbands than with their children. Their use of contradictory evaluative components in messages to their children (videotape analysis) would lend some support to the idea that they are either unwilling or unable to take an explicit and consistent stand with them. The meaning of these simultaneous, conflicting messages is not clear. They could reflect the mothers' uncertainty about their ability to make statements that would be accepted and complied with, resulting in incongruent, ineffectual communications. Or this conflict in evaluative meanings in different channels could represent the kind of contradictory messages described in the double-bind hypothesis, constricting children in a state of confusion. Yet a third alternative must be considered. These "conflicting" messages were recorded in the observed situation, and one part or channel of the communication might be aimed at presumed observers (a smiling face or a sweet voice, for example) with a separate component being directed toward the child (who would be supposed to get "his" message out of the mother's total communication, presumably recognizing it by its familiarity). In the same vein, part of the message (e.g., a sarcastic tone) might also be directed toward the father or other person in the room. In any case, some ambivalence, inconsistency, or social role playing may be reflected, in subtle but possibly important ways, in the R mothers' communication patterns. Further research is under way to clarify these alternatives.

PARENT→CHILD EFFECTS

The family environment of referred children was colored by much interpersonal devaluation, low levels of interpersonal interest and responsiveness, atypical parental role patterns, and extensive efforts on the part of all family members to exert control over each other. These were expressed in wide fluctuations of interpersonal activity and influence patterns. Such patterns constituted highly evaluative, affect-laden, and inconsistent stimuli for the children. In this sense R parents did not provide clearly defined role models that would facilitate identification and adequate social learning for either boys or girls. For the largely male child sample, there are indications that learning and modeling did take place (in terms of the father-child similarities in FARS, PBI, and videotapes). Unfortunately, however, the process seemed to involve the transmission of ineffectual behavior and fluctuating affect.

The observable consequences of the relatively low effectiveness of the father in the family may be reflected in the substantial impairment of the referred child's general effectiveness. This appeared in low physical education grades, relatively poor physical development and dexterity (PBI and TBI), difficulty in the communication task, and poor performance in carrying out a wide range of activities, as well as in his perceived high social negativity and low self-confidence (PBI, TBI, and FARS).

Similarly it seems possible that children do not flourish psychologically without the influence of a reasonably contented mother who exhibits satisfaction in her relationships and trust in her partner's competencies. For girls, there would seem to be inherent contradiction in modeling a maternal assumption of power that demonstrably brings little gratification.

There are other problems in addition to those of same-sex identification. Girls as well as boys depend on the father for learning many instrumental skills (Hetherington, 1965; Alkire, 1969). Our data suggest that, comparably, boys need the experience of having their emerging independence recognized in their interactions with a less controlling mother (FARS, PBI). Concurrently, in our R group, girls had little opportunity to learn to anticipate and support masculine competence in situations in which the mother usurped, competed for, or felt required to assume paternal power. Such inadequacies in the children's role exposures and experience would seem certain to lay the groundwork for the perpetuation of poor role performance when these children become adults.

In this sample of families, 46% of the R group contained no father in the home; in many other R families the father might be said to be psychologically absent in the sense that his expected roles were poorly exemplified by himself, and/or were often taken over by his wife. The importance of the effective presence of the father in instrumental roles seems evident from our results for control families. It is worth noting that the referred mothers appeared in our data to behave in much the same way with their children whether there was a father present or not. This suggests that an ineffective father may contribute little by his physical presence in the home.

In summary, the referred children were obviously distinguishable from the control children on all measures except the videotapes (where their deviant behaviors may have been temporarily "damped" by the presence of the observers). Their roles in the two sets of families, however, were not so clearly differentiated as were their fathers' behaviors—with which their own behavior was clearly closely associated, sometimes in apparent modeling or identification, sometimes in what appeared a reactive (or necessary) choice of an opposite style.

It has been noted that by the time children enter the third grade, the school setting has accumulated markedly feminine connotations for children, especially boys (Kagan, 1964). Since there was no father in the home for many more R than NR children, and since the pattern of psychological and behavioral involvement of the father seems critical in differentiating R and NR families, we speculate that a surfeit of feminine influence and a concomitant lack of masculine contact in the school environment is an important factor in the patterns of adjustment being reported, particularly for the boys, who comprise 81% of the sample. It is also surmised that the more dominant, controlling behavior reported for R mothers may trigger some antagonistic responses which these children suppress in the home but express more easily in interaction with the usually female schoolteacher.

It may be that the referred children were genetically or temperamentally impaired (relative to nonreferred children) and so themselves strongly influenced the behavior of the parents. Family interactions involve complex feedback patterns which make it impossible to identify discrete causes of behavior. However, the total interactional pattern of the two groups was observed to be quite different. The father's behavior and the relationships between parents indicate that relations with the child are only one component of larger patterns of family functioning.

These ongoing dysfunctional interactions in the family also suggest that it is not sufficient to postulate a simple social-learning theory interpretation of the results which emphasizes that learned dispositions to behave were primary determinants of behavior. There is no question that previously learned behaviors play an important role in affecting current behaviors; but children and parents seem locked in sets of ongoing behaviors and perceptions of each other which continuously influence what each person does.

PARENTAL PATTERNS

Our results are consonant with most of the family literature which generally reports poorly coordinated interactions and little effective leadership in families with troubled children. In our data the coalition between parents which Lidz (1967, p. 58) considers essential for a benign child rearing environment was absent from most referred families. Similarly, these families do not reflect the effective leadership patterns which Murrell and Stachowiak (1967) see as promoting children's successful adaptiveness. In their view, optimal leadership requires that parents have greater influence than children and that each parent should assume leadership in particular situations with the active cooperation and support of the spouse. This structured patterning of roles was evident in our control families but was distinctly absent in the referreds.

Most studies of leadership patterns in the family use some version of the Strodbeck technique (Winter & Ferreira, 1969, p. 99) in which the family must come to some consensus on issues about which they may disagree. The subject matter under discussion usually emphasizes concern about the expressive and emotional affairs of the family, such as children's rights and responsibilities. In our culture, according to Parsons and Bales (1954), these affairs are usually managed by the mother with the support of the father. In effectively functioning families, therefore, mothers should exercise leadership in this kind of discussion. Indeed, this seems to happen in the normal control families in several of the studies of this type (Murrell & Stachowiak, 1967; Hutchinson, 1969; Bodin, 1969).* In the families with disturbed children, however, as Murrell and Stachowiak suggest, fathers often seem to compete with the mother for the emotional-expressive leadership with little evidence of any instrumental leadership on their part. Thus the families of disturbed children often lack the type of leadership that the fathers are supposed to provide. Our families' clinic behavior seems generally related to this kind of family process: the father intruded excessively into the mother's domain (videotapes), without providing strength and leadership in the more instrumental functions of the family (FARS, PBI, Family Task).

Concomitantly, the R mother, in our data, often accepted or assumed paternal prerogatives and expressed her lack of confidence in her husband in unmistakable terms.

The basic question, therefore, would seem to be not whether the mother or the father is more powerful in the family. It is rather focused on the areas in which leadership is exercised by each parent and the manner in which each supports the other within his or her domain.

Qualitatively, interactions within the R families seemed characterized by much tension, irritation, and ignoring behavior. Parental responsibilities seemed onerous and unrewarding. There was little evidence that familial relationships were a source of pleasure, comfort, or security. (Again it is emphasized that there was no lack of love or concern manifested.) The picture is one of parents (especially fathers) who do not feel able to do what they consider is expected or required of them, and spouses who mutually reinforce feelings of parental inadequacy.

Though we have no way of characterizing the personal adequacy of the parents, our findings are not inconsistent with previous reports about the characteristics of parents with troubled children. For example, both Liverant (1959) and Goodstein and Rowley (1961) found consistently greater maladjustment in the parents of disturbed than of nondisturbed children. But our data suggest that the critical problems are deficiencies in the areas of personal self-confidence, role security, and interpersonal trust. Moreover, any sense of familial relationships as a potential source of personal gratifica-

* It is difficult to draw conclusions regarding leadership or power in families from the results of Strodbeck-type studies because (a) the results tend to vary, perhaps due to the variety of measures of power used (e.g., number of words spoken by a member, the choice of the individual solution adopted by the group); (b) there is no independent criterion for the measure of "power" reported in these studies; and (c) the Strodbeck technique itself represents one particular contrived type of interaction which seems an insufficient basis for generalization.

tion seems consistently absent. The interpersonal arena was described as a source of mutual pleasure and support by nonreferred families, but referred families depicted their relationships as weighted with intolerable responsibility and clouded with threat to the self.

Parenthetically, we suspect that noteworthy differences between the two sets of family data which have yet to be analyzed are manifest in the different kinds of humor utilized in control versus referred families.

SUMMARY OF R/NR CHARACTERISTICS AND PATTERNS

Our results for referred families depict a highly consistent family style, consisting of an overall evaluative aura with predominantly negative perceptions and interactions. Interpersonal anxiety and negativism are expressed by all family members, with personal insecurity a particular difficulty of many fathers. There is no effective organizing structure within the family group. The usual parental role differentiations are confused, with conflictual efforts to control the spouse and child demonstrated by each parent. The father fails to assume leadership in instrumental tasks and involves himself instead in competing with the mother or complying with her demand that he feel responsible for the emotional management of the family. Conversely the mother attributes a low level of competence to her husband, describes a dominant role for herself, and assumes many of the normally paternal instrumental functions.

The father's dissatisfaction and discomfort with his resulting ineffectual status is apparent in his easily provoked emotional reactivity and his persistent but shifting efforts to exert interpersonal impact and to gain status.

The mother's uneasy reaction to her perhaps tenuous position is more subtly reflected in her self-perception as more passive on the FARS than she is seen by others; in her conflicting messages (her inconsistencies across channel components within messages to her child); and most of all in her lack of expressed pleasure in her life situation. The referred mothers do not rate or report themselves as gratified in their interpersonal relationships, either with their husbands or with the adult community. The psychological closeness and the relatively high amount of the activity they claim with their children suggests a compensatory involvement with them that is related to their unsatisfactory adult relationships. This seems especially likely since their descriptions of their mutual interactions with the children also seem generally negative in content and tone.

If the above interpretations are correct, referred fathers in our study demonstrated that they are of little help to their children in learning to handle their environment. They fail both as examples and as leaders who should create and maintain a family climate that encourages competence with tasks and effectiveness with people. The R mothers contribute to this outcome when they fail to provide support for the fathers' efforts. They further exacerbate problems when they assume the fathers' prerogatives, either by intention or as a consequence of paternal default.

These results suggest that where personal roles are poorly defined and assimilated, interpersonal relationships will be poorly articulated and unreliable. Children from such interpersonal backgrounds will have difficulty in acquiring definition for themselves and developing secure expectations of others. Implications seem abundant for the transfer of interpersonal difficulties as such children leave the home and attempt to form new social relations in the world outside. In their early efforts to adapt to elementary school, for example, these children had run into conspicuous difficulties.

Socioeconomic Level Differences (Referred and Nonreferred Groups Combined.)

For the parents, the major findings were that verbal sophistication, including the effectiveness of verbal information sharing, decreased in the order of Hi > Mid > Lo SEL. This pattern was found for both verbal intelligence estimates (FRPV) and performance in the communication task, and was not related to referred-nonreferred categories. Accordingly, different levels of verbal sophistication within families do not by themselves appear to be major factors differentiating the chronically troubled from the more effectively operating families. Problems of communication, if they are important, must be identified in more complex patterns of mutual understanding, not simply on the level of verbal effectiveness. It must be emphasized that these SEL findings refer only to *verbal* communication, since visual clues were excluded from the communication task.

Additional SEL effects were found in the fathers' and mothers' responses to the Behavior Inventories. Hi SEL fathers tended to consider their children as more affectionate and more responsive to them than did fathers in either the Mid or Lo SEL groups. And their children rated them as more socially competent than did lower SEL children.

Lo SEL mothers described themselves as angry and frustrated in comparison to the reports of Hi SEL mothers. They saw themselves as the decision makers in the family and were highly dissatisfied with their physical environments, including home and neighborhood. This effect seems related to the realistic economic, social, and psychological problems faced by the Lo SEL mothers.

There were no significant interactions between SEL and R/NR categories for findings related to parents. In terms of an overview of findings related to these major categorizations, however, a number of factors seem to have been involved in the reported familial difficulties. (1) One is the single-parent situation. For any single parent at any SEL, the sense of total responsibility (economic, cultural, and psychological) seemed a tremendous burden. The family composition differences reported in Chapter 2 are exemplified throughout the study. (2) Second is socioeconomic level itself. It would seem evident that some basic level of social and vocational security is needed to reduce personal anxieties and increase time and potential for interpersonal gratification. Beyond such levels, however, additional security does not ensure more effective interpersonal functioning. (3) There is the question of the clarity and consistency with which parental responsibilities are allocated and shared between R and NR parents. Our four sets of family data all reflect much greater structure in parental behaviors in control families. (4) Finally there is the adequacy with which each parent fulfills his or her own role within the family, in his own eyes and in the evaluations of other family members. It is in this area that the focus on the R/NR differences in fathers' behavior became paramount. It may be that the R fathers are individually somehow less adequate than are their control counterparts. It may also be that their patterns of adequacy simply do not fit present cultural stereotypes of what paternal behavior should be.

Most of these factors are compounded in the case of Lo SEL R mothers. These women, about half of whom were single parents, were demonstrably more dissatisfied with their life situation than higher SEL mothers (PBI), whether or not there was a father in the home.

More detailed empirical analysis of role functioning within the family, and across SELs, is required for a better understanding of the genesis and maintenance of troubled behavior in children; but particularly for children who are having difficulty in the elementary school setting, our findings for (1) the importance of an active, involved father in the home, and (2) the integrally related roles of two parents in the home seem significant at any SEL.

Referral Category Differences

In the family data, only the detailed analyses of the videotapes indicate systematic relationships between the type of problem exhibited by the child at school and specific characteristics of family behavior. These results suggest that children with predominant problems of aggression in school are most likely to have fathers who appear unfriendly and dictatorial while interacting with their families in the clinic and mothers who, in the same situation, convey contradictory evaluative meanings in the different channels (e.g., voice, content) of their communications to the children. Fathers who were highly inconsistent in their expressive range (being highly positive and/or highly negative) tended to have children who manifested attention control problems at school. Fathers who were exceedingly talkative in the observed family interactions had children who were socially withdrawn at school. It is important to note that it was possible to identify those differentiations only when recorded verbal *and* nonverbal data were available for detailed and repeated review.

CHILDREN AT HOME AND SCHOOL

Referred—Nonreferred Differences

Parents and teachers essentially agreed on the variables which differentiated R and NR children. On the Adjective Rating Scales, R children were rated consistently more unfavorably than the NR children on both Positive and Negative Social Impact. On the Behavior Inventories both adult groups agreed in characterizing the R children as less socially effective, more hostile and destructive, more withdrawn, and less task oriented than the NR children. These findings are in general agreement with results reported by Cowen, Huser, Beach, and Rappaport (1970) who found that parents' perceptions were systematically related to teachers' judgments of children's adjustment. In that study also, parents and teachers agreed on the particular behaviors differentiating R and NR children. The similarity in perceptions indicates that the disturbing behaviors which led to referral were not restricted to the school setting, so that a simple situational concept of troubled behavior is not tenable.

Project observers also reflected the expected R/NR differences on the negativity factor in both the classroom and playground ratings. This additional confirmation indicates that the initial R/NR classification was not due to teacher bias in their assessment of the children.

There was one exception to the pattern in which an evaluative difference favoring the control children was reported significantly and consistently in all settings and by all raters. This was the rating of children's videotaped behavior in the family room. There the perceived differentiation was in terms of the fact that the referred children's behavior was usually affectively colored, appearing either very positive or very negative, not in terms of overall differences in positive versus negative qualities. This finding suggests that the condition of being observed had a pronounced effect on children, just as it had on all mothers and on referred fathers. It apparently increased tension, triggering expressive reactions; but it simultaneously reduced the R children's overtly negative behaviors, just as it may have increased R mothers' and fathers' evidences of positive, approving expressions. Both seem indications of specific situational effects on behavior. (The referred children's ability to curb their negative behavior when they feel it dangerous or inappropriate is perhaps noteworthy in itself. It may also reflect a situationally induced decrease in parental actions and interactions that serve to stimulate the children's problem behaviors.)

Several relationships between child and father behaviors were also reported. Correlations between their manifestations of highly expressive behaviors, talkativeness, and directing behavior all imply that at this age level the child models the father directly. This seems especially important since there were no comparable similarities found for child and mother behaviors. It would seem that the child's interpersonal style is quite similar to the father's, especially in the activity and directing dimensions and in his degree and patterns of emotional expressiveness.

In their self-perceptions, the referred children tended to agree with the predominantly unfavorable perceptions others had of them. Their self-ratings (FARS) were consistently more negative than the nonreferred children's self-ratings, and the referred children expected to be seen unfavorably by both parents. The referred children thus were quite aware of how others saw them and, in their self-ratings, shared the adults' unfavorable view of them.

Socioeconomic Level Differences

For the child, no consistent or replicated SEL main effects were obtained on any of the instruments except the graduated decline in grades and FRPV IQ with SEL.

Interrelationships between membership in referred and nonreferred groups and different socioeconomic levels were found only in the school data. Hi and Lo SEL referred children, by and large, were referred for similar reasons. For both, the number of cases in each referral category deceased in the order of Aggression > Hyperactivity > Attention Control > Social Withdrawal. For the Mid SEL, on the other hand, the order was Attention Control > Social Withdrawal > Hyperactivity > Aggression (Chapter 2). Interestingly, the Behavior Inventories of teachers in the Lo SEL schools indicate that they saw these referred children as socially quite effective, whereas they considered the nonreferred Lo SEL children quiet and highly conforming. Teachers in Hi SEL schools generally rated their referred pupils as more aggressive than did teachers in lower SEL schools, and considered their Hi SEL referred children as particularly aggressive and disturbing. In teachers' Positive Impact ratings, the differences between the referred and nonreferred children were largest for the Hi SEL group, and smallest for the Lo SEL. Mid SEL referred children were seen as largely conforming, manifesting a preponderance of problems associated with social withdrawal, somatic problems, anxiety, and the like.

Although Hi and Lo SEL children were often referred for similar types of problems, the social environments in the schools were quite different for these two groups. Both Hi and Lo SEL schools were in socioeconomically and ethnically homogeneous areas. Almost all of the children in Lo SEL schools were black and from poor families. Almost all of the children in the three Hi SEL schools were white and from relatively high income families. The preponderance of teachers in both sets of schools were Mid SEL. It was our impression that the Hi SEL schools from which the sample was drawn encouraged children to express themselves freely and therefore tolerated a much wider range of behaviors (including aggression) than did the Mid and Lo SEL schools. Thus, although the Hi SEL children showed a high level of socially negative behavior, both in teachers' and in observers' ratings, it seems that there was a higher tolerance in these schools for such behavior. By contrast, the Lo SEL school personnel usually expressed a great deal of concern about their problems in controlling the children's aggressive behavior. Our impressions were that the Lo SEL children's higher activity levels, often interpreted as aggressive, resulted partly from the social and cultural patterns from which these children came and partly from the expectations by school personnel (e.g., expect Lo SEL children to be impulsive and aggressive, Hi SEL children to be expressive and assertive). Similarly, teachers of Hi SEL children often ascribed their referred children's deviance to parental failure to provide structure for the child and to channel his assertiveness, while teachers of Lo SEL children usually complained about what they considered parents' lack of interest or motivation to control their children. We do not, however, have any data relevant to these observations.

Referral Category Differences

The relationships between the child's referral category and parental behavior have already been presented.

Most school ratings also differentiated children in the different referral categories. On adjective ratings, teachers regarded the aggressive and hyperactive children as more socially negative relative to the average child than the children in other referral categories. In contrast, children classified as socially withdrawn were rated as less negative than average. In the Teacher Behavior Inventory, the aggressive children were seen as nonconforming but as more effective leaders than other referred children. Project observers' adjective ratings essentially confirmed the teachers' ratings. These coinciding views suggest that aggressive children were referred largely because of their behavior in the classroom rather than on the playground, where their high self-confidence supported the teachers' belief in their interpersonal effectiveness with peers. Possibly the same qualities that foster effectiveness with peers are an obstacle to smooth relationships with adults. Aggression, successful on the playground, may be maladaptive in the classroom.

Hyperactive children were observed to behave like the aggressive children in the classroom. On the playground, however, they appeared unfriendly, without the constructive leadership observed in aggressive children. Socially withdrawn children, as expected, showed relatively low positive impact on others but also received relatively high ratings for negative impact. Attention control children tended to be given lowest scores by observers in almost all of their ratings, indicating little involvement in any activities. In a sense, they appear to show responses of massive avoidance. It seems possible that the specific requirements of the learning process which predominates in the school setting are somehow particularly difficult for these children, and are in some way especially incompatible with their abilities and behavior patterns. This speculation obviously introduces room for a range of difficulties associated with temperamental, cognitive, or physical differences inherent in individual children's makeup. The environmental emphasis reported in our work is meant to be literally that: an emphasis for heuristic purposes, not a statement of an all-encompassing generality about children's problem behaviors. Such difficulties obviously have individual as well as environmental bases. Group situations (like classrooms) inevitably highlight such individual deviations and idiosyncracies.

THE SCHOOL SETTING

Almost all the referred children had been a source of concern to the school and to parents for some time before referral. School records, as well as our interviews with teachers, indicated considerable variability in teachers' abilities to deal with these children. Occasionally, a child's previous teacher could not understand why a child was seen as troubled, indicating that the class and the school environment can suppress, temporarily eliminate, or conversely, accentuate children's troubled behaviors. But most usually troubled children's problems seemed to increase and become compounded over time.

Analyses of the family data have so far revealed some findings relating patterns of family functioning to the child's predominant referral problem; most of these appear in the videotape analyses. Taken as a whole, our empirical findings and anecdotal impressions lead us to conclude that referral problems identified at school result largely from the interaction of these individual patterns with the sociocultural stresses in the specific school setting. The specificity of "symptom" designation to particular settings is quite consonant with the results reported by others (e.g., Speer, 1971). As Speer notes, " . . . we can begin by frankly acknowledging (a) the role of situational variables (including adult behavior) in precipitating children's "symptomatic" behavior, (b) the marked individual differences in adults' tolerance for, and sensitivities and reaction to, various kinds of behavior, and (c) the marked individual differences in adults' interpretations, evaluations, and labeling of children's behaviors" (p. 227). *Our conclusion at this time is that until the kind of behavioral data contained in the videotapes of families becomes available for the analysis of schoolroom and playground interactions, we will not be able to identify many of the specific referents for children's behavioral reactions at school.*

CONCLUSIONS

The results reported in this section suggest two major sets of conclusions:

1. Almost all the children who functioned adequately in the school setting came from families in which fathers and mothers had differentiated, complementary, and stable familial roles. Referred children, in contrast, experienced chronic turmoil in their families and usually did not have parents who assumed, or consistently maintained, the culturally expected roles. Accordingly, behavior that is seen by the school as effective seems to emerge within an interpersonal environment in which children observe and develop behavior patterns and expectations which facilitate pleasurable, complementary functioning with others. We interpret the findings as indicating that, to the extent to which different types of behavior (e.g., expressive, instrumental) are required for effective interpersonal functioning, there must be persons in the child's living environment who consistently exemplify them. If important functions are divided along male-female lines, then males and females may be required to enact these roles vis-à-vis the child. Models of culturally adaptive behavior are needed not only to help children form sexual and other identities, but also to serve as a continuing monitoring and teaching environment, at least throughout the elementary-school years.

In the view propounded in this report, the child does not simply model behaviors by imitating others, but experiments continuously in his interactions with adults. The adult is a stimulus for the child, and vice versa. The child's own adaptiveness emerges from the give and take of such ongoing interactions. If this is so it would seem that situations in which many children relate to one adult, or where many adults relate to the same child, cannot easily be substituted for family-like settings. For example, nursery or elementary schools usually involve a woman with a number of children. Although these experiences can be extremely valuable in helping children to acquire basic cognitive and interpersonal skills, both from the teacher and peers, they take place in an essentially ad hoc group for the child. Also, since the teacher's relationship with the child is relatively temporary for him, that is, limited in place (classroom, playground), time, and function (e.g., to encourage learning in a group of children), she cannot encourage the range or closeness of interactions that can occur in more nuclear group relationships, in which continuing processes are consistently repeated in myriad variations.

2. Although our analyses have yielded some information as to how patterns of family behavior influence symptom selection in the schools, our school data did not include the behavioral records which permit the detailed and repeated scrutiny necessary to define specific stimulus patterns for children's different reactions. As far as we can determine from our data, the blend between the child's interpersonal environment at school, his sociocultural background, and specific parental patterns all appear to be involved in the resultant *type* of problem that children manifest at school. For children who lack an appropriate father model, the predominance of female teachers may accentuate the problem of role appropriate socialization. And schools may contribute substantially to children's difficulties by not providing a cultural and interpersonal context within which pupils can experience comfort and success. The resultant failure to develop confidence in self, and trust and confidence in others, further compounds children's difficulties since it interferes with their ability to acquire the cognitive tools needed for effective functioning in the larger society.

However, whatever the school program, it is doubtful that school training can be successful without substantial cooperation between the school and the home. Cognitive and other skills learned in school cannot become useful to the children unless their home environment provides support and stimulation for the exercise of relevant behavior. Thus what is learned in the school must be pertinent, or potentially pertinent, to the children's psychosocial environment and must involve their daily living contexts.

For children from poor and otherwise disadvantaged minority group backgrounds, schools and communities are often far apart in values, objectives, and practices. Recent efforts to relate schools to community needs may help children more with cognitive and social learning than could specific educational reforms carried out in the school alone. Our results indicate a need to focus increased attention on the structure and viability of primary social reference groups as the most important determinants of children's behavior during the elementary-school years. Schools must tie into these initial familial environments and build upon their strengths.

A final comment within this segment of our report is addressed to the generalized disregard shown by most adults for their own nonverbal behavior. Parents and teachers use lectures and verbal strictures as if these were the only input they give to the child. In hours of observation of family interactions and teacher behavior in the classroom, we experienced the massive outpouring of adult verbiage to which the child is expected to listen attentively and acceptingly. At the same time, he is flooded by additional sets of nonverbal cues, of most of which parents and teachers seem genuinely unaware. The child apparently has, as a major developmental task, to learn to make this artificial differentiation: he is supposed to respond primarily to adults' words, not to the other channels of communication in which the words are embedded.

The extent to which verbalization has been accepted as the equivalent of total communication by most adults is interesting in retrospect, especially in the light of the importance of our nonverbal data in discriminating between poorly and well-functioning families. The implications for self-deception, poor communication, and disturbed interpersonal relationships inherent in this generalized social convention are profound. The fact that this same equivalence has characterized the social institution of psychotherapy is reflected in Part II.

PART TWO

Treatments

CHAPTER 7

The Design for the Comparison of Treatments

At the time this study was planned, the most widespread means of treatment for children's problems emphasized psychotherapy for the child and professional counseling for the parents. In order to evaluate the effectiveness of our Information Feedback intervention, therefore, we planned a comparison between the outcomes of "Feedback" with these two standard approaches. The three treatments differed in several basic characteristics: the focus of the intervention, the role of the clinician, the definition of the problem, and the type of change process believed to be involved.*

CHARACTERISTICS OF THE THREE TREATMENTS

In *Child Therapy* the therapist dealt with the child directly, even though parents were often seen adjunctively and some therapists occasionally saw the entire family group. The therapist's role was to provide acceptance and emotional support, enabling the child to learn to experience his own feelings, and in some cases to expand the child's understanding of his experience. The relationship with the therapist was considered the essential medium for providing acceptance, insight, and opportunity for change. This treatment, essentially based on versions of psychoanalytic theory and addressed to the child's psychodynamic processes, involved the notion of disordered function within the child, albeit with recognition that many problems were initiated by or related to familial and environmental factors. The effectiveness of the child's coping behavior was seen as depending to a large extent on the maturity, flexibility, and integration of his psychological states, that is, feelings, motives, and attitudes. Treatment of his psychological characteristics was therefore expected to improve his coping effectiveness.

---

* Portions of this material are also reported in Love, Kaswan, and Bugental, 1972. © 1972 by the American Psychological Association and reprinted by permission.

In *Parent Counseling,* the parents met with a clinician whose role was that of an understanding, interested authority who provided expert advice, indicating how parents might change their behavior and expectations with respect to the child. Counselors who use this type of intervention tend to assume that children's problems are due largely to parents' deficient knowledge about the kinds of parental behavior likely to assist the psychological development of their children. Accordingly, a major task in such intervention is to suggest parental behaviors that are likely to be corrective of problems. Such instruction as to amount and kind of "parenting" has traditionally characterized the American child guidance movement.

Information Feedback involved both the family and school personnel in looking at the child's interpersonal environment as reflected in the assessments described in the preceding section. Both parents and teachers were recipients of feedback, though the main focus was on the parents. In this view, the child's problems were postulated to reflect his inability to adapt to overly complex, incongruous, or insensitive facets of his interpersonal environment. The significant adults who figured in these environments were assumed to be unaware of the impact of their verbal and nonverbal communications on the child and the complex of contradictory messages and expectations to which he was supposed to adapt. In this approach, a relatively impersonal consultant offered the adults his feedback materials for their own scrutiny, and consciously avoided promoting their dependency on his support or advice. New information, or old information in new and salient form, was presented to stimulate the client's own problem-solving and change-producing efforts. This approach emphasized the importance of the perceptions and behavior of significant adults in determining children's behavior, and the role of interpersonal information in promoting attitude and behavior change. The information was obtained directly through the adults' own observation, not through interpretations or suggestions offered by a clinician.

A basic contrast was thus embodied in the *type of professional relationship* posited for clinicians in each of the three treatments. This variable seemed important to incorporate since its role in the treatment process had so far defied clear specification. The original concept of a therapeutic relationship as the primary agent of change in psychotherapeutic process has proved to be hard to codify. It is not necessarily distinguishable from other kinds of relationships (Schofield, 1964; Cartwright, 1968) and its successful utilization is not restricted to professional therapists (Knapp & Holzberg, 1964; Poser, 1966; Carkhuff, 1968). Indeed some clinicians seem unable to create and utilize the relationship effectively (Truax, 1963; Betz, 1967), and some patients improve without benefit of any relationship at all (Frank, 1963). For these reasons, the type of relationship was a central variable in this study. The three treatments contrast the understanding, empathic therapist, the helpful advice-giving counselor, and the relatively impersonal consultant who collects and "feeds back" current interpersonal information. This variation in clinician's role seemed to epitomize and incorporate the other differences in the treatments: the focus of the intervention, the definition of the problem, and the type of change process believed to be involved.

METHODOLOGY

In planning the comparison of these three treatments a number of methodological considerations emphasized in the literature on research on psychotherapy were included: (1) a heterogeneous sample of families and schools with respect to SEL; (2) standardized referral and clinical procedures; (3) random assignment of cases to treatments; (4) objective outcome criteria; and (5) follow-up measures.

Range of Socioeconomic Level of Clients

Our interest in the relationships between sociocultural factors and a number of family, school, and treatment variables made comparisons associated with socioeconomic level an important aspect of our work. Consequently we drew on the widest range of socioeconomic levels that was (a) geographically feasible and (b) would provide samples large enough to permit statistical comparisons. Within each level we included as wide a range of children's difficulties as could be found in public-school settings.

Standardized Referral and Clinical Procedures

To ensure that all families would come to the clinic with a reasonably common orientation and set of expectations, we involved principals, teachers, and counselors from all our 10 schools in group meetings in which a general understanding of the clinic and its services was developed. School personnel used this information as a basis for referral discussions with all families. This combined school-and-project group also developed a common framework for selection, observation, and referral procedures to be followed in all schools.

The referral criteria were: (1) children should be between 8 and 12 years of age; (2) they should be manifesting severe social, behavioral, or emotional problems; (3) the school should have exhausted its own helping resources; (4) children should be receiving no current professional help, and have had none in the recent past; (5) the presence of a "learning problem" was immaterial but all children should be in regular classrooms. Each school was given a quota of referrals for the 2 years during which cases could be accepted for treatment within the project. Individual teachers could refer only one child a year.

Referrals were determined by a consensus between a child's teacher, counselor, and principal. One of these then contacted the parents to determine their interest in having the child seen at the university. Parents were told that members of the UCLA psychology staff were currently working with children whose problems were similiar to their child's. If parents were interested in exploring the possibility of some kind of treatment, they signed a consent slip permitting the school counselor to send information about their child to the clinic.

All referred families were offered treatment. When referral information was received from the school, parents were contacted and offered an appointment. They were told that, at least for the first visit, the entire family unit (everyone currently living in the home, whether relative or friend) would have to come in. Fees for service were set on a sliding scale based on income and number of dependents, but it was made clear that inability to pay was not a basis for exclusion from service. In instances of financial or geographic problems, transportation by university car was provided. Every effort was made to equalize opportunity for utilizing project services. No advance information was given about any specific type of treatment. Parents were informed that problems could be approached in a variety of ways and that the treatment available for their child's problem would be described in the initial interview.

Before their first appointment, each family received a standard letter describing the training and research functions of the clinic. This included observation and recording in all clinic rooms, our ongoing efforts to develop new treatment methods, and the fact that some services were provided by graduate students under staff supervision. Families were invited to call the clinic or raise questions about any of these procedures at any time.

Upon arriving at the clinic, after it had been ascertained that they had received and read the letter, all families had the same initial experience of being observed and videotaped in the "family" room. Beyond this point, procedures differed according to the treatment to which the family had been assigned. The 30 Information Feedback and 29 control (NR) families participated in all four techniques designed to provide feedback data (FARS, PBI, Communication Task, and videotaping). Half of the 28 Parent Counseling and 33 Child Therapy families took part in the FARS, PBI, and Communication Task. The restriction of these measures to half of the families receiving the standard treatments was designed to permit evaluation of possible effects of experiencing these experimental techniques without feedback.

Following the initial measures obtained in the first appointment, an interview was conducted by the clinician with whom the family would be working thereafter. From this point, each therapist or parent counselor proceeded as he would in his own practice, with the exception that he explicitly set a prescribed maximum limit to the number of appointments treatment would cover. All three interventions were time limited, as outlined later in this chapter. Though the Child Therapists or Parent Counselors had only the school referral information supplied them initially, they were free to seek further information from schools or other agencies. These clinicians did not know the design or purpose of the project and no research data were available to them. For example, they did not observe the family or see adjective rating scales, behavior inventories, or other measures used by the Information Feedback consultants as the core of their feedback procedures.

All "feedback" consultants followed semistructured interview formats and focused their sessions on collection and feedback of the interpersonal material they were gathering through the videotapes, ratings, questionnaires, and family communication tasks. Their procedures are detailed in Chapter 10.

A flow chart which summarizes the standard procedures for processing all cases can be found in Appendix A, pp. 249–250).

Random Assignment of Cases to Treatments

The importance of utilizing random assignment to treatment conditions has been discussed widely (e.g., Ford and Urban, 1967) but rarely implemented in situations dealing with human problems. The inclusion of this important methodological procedure was made possible by the flexibility and research orientation of all the clinicians and school personnel who worked with us in this study. Since all treatments were seen as potentially useful for all cases, we could utilize random assignment and let the results determine the characteristics of children and families for which each intervention would prove optimally helpful. Because referrals came from different schools at different rates, occasional corrections were made to equalize socioeconomic levels within treatment groups (e.g., social class representation was equalized within both Year I and Year II groups of families). Occasional scheduling problems necessitated assignment to a treatment for which there was an available clinician as there was no overlap among the clinicians providing the three types of service. Apart from a few nonrecurring instances, however, cases were assigned automatically to treatment groups in rotation, without regard to the characteristics of the case.

The Use of Objective Outcome Measures

Studies over the last two decades have reflected the difficulty of demonstrating that people "improve" as the result of psychological treatment (e.g., Eysenck, 1967), especially in terms of objective criteria (e.g., Paul, 1966). Outcome studies of psychotherapeutic work with children have been relatively few, but clear-cut indications of positive outcomes have been hard to find (e.g., Levitt, 1963, 1957). Earlier focus on psychodynamic variables entailed reliance on verbal reports of the participants in treatment, a criterion subject to possible bias from a number of sources. More recent attention to behavioral variables permits more objective appraisal of change (e.g., Moustakas & Schalock, 1955; Seeman, Barry, & Ellinwood, 1964), and the trend toward measurement of behavior changes manifested outside the treatment situation (e.g., Schulman, Shoemaker, & Moelis, 1962) further limits sources of bias. In this study we used repeated judgments of children's behavior in the school setting as basic criteria for evaluating the outcomes of treatment supplied in the clinic. These included school grades and observers' standardized ratings of children's behavior in interactions with teachers and peers. Neither of these measures should reflect any systematic bias which could influence evaluations of treatment outcome. Other measures, such as ratings by family members and teachers and changes in recorded behavior in the clinic, were used only as supplementary measures of outcome, since they seemed more susceptible to possible bias.

SCHOOL GRADES

Though the reliability and validity of grades leave much to be desired, they seemed to provide the most objective, independent, and nonreactive measure available for comparing children's changes across all schools and all treatment groups. Since the children were referred specifically for behavioral difficulties at school, indices of school adjustment seemed appropriate criteria for assessing desired behavior change. In addition, although the referral criteria were set up to specify behavioral disturbances in children other than learning difficulties per se, approximately 80% of the referred children were also considered to have some difficulty in achievement areas. For these reasons, grades seem to reflect the child's overall functional competence and comfort in the school environment.

In order to get information on the child's prereferral performance, we obtained all recorded grades, both achievement and conduct, from three semesters previous to project participation to the end of the follow-up intervals beyond termination dates for all cases. For each child we averaged all grades at each point in time to obtain a composite number reflecting both conduct and achievement (see Appendix A, pp. 233–234).

Since the Information Feedback intervention involved the child's current teacher in some interaction with the consultant, criterion grades used for outcome measures were those obtained at the conclusion of the *third* semester following intake. By this time all children were in different grades with different teachers (and over 25% were in different schools). Therefore no bias should be reflected in the school grades criterion which would favor any particular type of intervention.

SCHOOL OBSERVER RATINGS

As described in Appendix A, p. 248, children's behavior at school was rated by trained judges. Initial ratings were made of referred, nonreferred, and an additional group of randomly identified children, with the raters unaware of any child's classification or of the specific purpose of any ratings. In the classroom the child was rated separately on his interactions with the teacher and with his peers. The third rating was of his behavior with peers on the playground. Ratings were made with the adjective scales and results are reported in terms of the two factors which emerged in all analyses of adjective ratings: (a) the Negative Social Impact and (b) the Positive Social Impact attributed to the interpersonal behaviors being judged.

Though both basic outcome criteria, school grades and observer's behavior ratings, are subjective judgments, the fact that they are quite independent of each other should add credibility, to whatever extent the results vary together.

FOLLOW-UP PROCEDURES

The project design incorporated follow-up visits to the clinic for all available families at intervals of approximately 6, 12, and 24 months after termination of the treatment series. Apart from the contribution as follow-up data, it was anticipated that the posttreatment sessions would have a "booster" impact on all groups. Others have expressed similar hopes for follow-up sessions (Bellak & Small, 1967; Glasser, 1967).

In most instances, it was possible to have the original clinician see the family for at least the first follow-up interview. These sessions at the clinic included a repetition of whatever measures the family had experienced on their original visit (including the videotaping of the family in the family room) and an interview conducted by their previous clinician. When he was not available, the interview was conducted by a clinician who utilized the same type of intervention the family had received and who had familiarized himself with the material in the family case folder.

At the same follow-up intervals, current school grades, teacher reports, and behavior observations were collected in the school settings. The fact that schools were not in session during summer months made for some variation in the timing of this procedure, but this was constant across all groups. As an additional follow-up, grades for all children who could be located (80%) were obtained 2 years following the end of the clinic contacts.

FORMATS OF THE THREE TREATMENTS

Child Psychotherapy

For reasons of time and cost, psychotherapy had to be limited to 20 sessions or less. We recognized that many clinicians would consider this an inadequate number of sessions to produce change even though it far exceeded in duration the national averages of actual psychotherapeutic treatment for either children or adults (Eiduson, 1968). This time limitation was also designed to make the child therapy group comparable to the experimental group receiving Information Feedback (whose procedures were designed originally to cover 12 weeks). In discussions during early project planning, child therapists indicated that during the initial weeks they would be likely to have separate interviews with the parents and the child within a given week; on this basis 20 sessions over a 12-week interval seemed to provide a roughly equivalent amount of professional contact for the feedback and the therapy interventions. In actual practice these time limitations were in effect only for Year I cases. Completion of the Information Feedback procedures did not require the 12 sessions planned, so in Year II both interventions were shortened: Child Therapy to 12 sessions, Information Feedback to 8.

Effective treatment for Child Therapy was expected to be related closely to the experience of the clinician. Therefore, except for one case carried in each year by an advanced graduate student, all children were seen by experienced, practicing therapists from the Los Angeles professional community who had specialized in child work. They were selected from the roster of a local professional organization on the basis of experience, reputation, and their belief that short-term child oriented psychotherapy was an effective method of treating children's behavior disorders. Therapists were paid at standard professional hourly rates. All treatment was carried out at the UCLA Psychology Clinic.

In the first year one highly experienced child therapist carried all cases except the one seen by a graduate student. In order not to base our results on the effectiveness of one practitioner, second year cases were assigned to six other professional clinicians, thus permitting an evaluation of treatment outcomes for one therapist, as compared with the outcomes of six others. In making this decision, we blurred the comparison between the two years by altering two variables (number of maximum hours, 20 reduced to 12, and number of clinicians, one increased to six). The usual dilemmas of rigor versus reality were with us.

Parent Counseling

The counseling services were similar to those offered by many family service or Parent-Teacher Association clinics. Focusing on the immediate situation, the clinician used interviews and tests to identify the child's major problems. On the basis of this assessment he counseled one or both parents, usually giving interpretations, suggestions, or advice based on child rearing principles and his own clinical experience. The treatment was designed to be quite brief, usually involving four or five sessions.

In the first year, service to the parents was supplied by two psychology and two social work graduate students under social work supervision. In Year II, all Parent Counseling services were supplied by six experienced social workers (through contract with a local professional organization, at current professional rates). All counselors were committed to this approach. During both years the interview with the child, and any testing deemed appropriate, was done by psychology graduate students with staff supervision.

Information Feedback

Information Feedback involved the families in two or three sessions in which interpersonal information was gathered through the four project measures described in the preceding section. Then the parents and, at parental option, the children had four or five sessions devoted to viewing and discussing the materials derived from all the family and school measures. Similarities and differences were presented largely through visual media (e.g., superimposed graphs and profiles of individuals' ratings, questionnaire responses, and the like). Such visual presentation left participants free to identify and choose the material that seemed important or change-worthy to them. School personnel (always including the child's teacher), attended one session at the clinic, viewing the information about their own interaction with the child. The family was not present at this meeting but within the limits specified in parental permission, representative data about the child's family were included. A final meeting was held at the school with parents and school personnel (teacher, principal, counselor, or other concerned staff). The consultant was present as a resource person but the meeting was set up and conducted by the principal. The purpose of this meeting was to foster mutual discussion and planning between the significant adults from both of the critical settings in the child's life.

Consultants were members of the UCLA Psychology Clinic staff. The authors worked with cases during both years; four other clinic staff members and four graduate students carried the rest of the cases. As discussed above, the maximum number of sessions for Year I was 12, and 8 for Year II.

FAMILY AND CHILD CHARACTERISTICS WITHIN TREATMENT GROUPS

The distribution of family and child characteristics within different treatment groups appears in Table 1. This table shows that socioeconomic level was fairly equally distributed across treatment groups. Efforts had been made to ensure this distribution for each of the two years of case processing since the interaction between social class and type of treatment was of major interest. Family composition was similar for the three groups except for the smaller number of two-parent families receiving Parent Counseling. Referral Categories were not distributed evenly among treatments: Aggressiveness

Table 1. Family and Child Characteristics Within Treatment Groups: Total R

	Information Feedback	Parent Counseling	Child Therapy	Total
Socioeconomic level				
High	6	8	7	21
Middle	16	13	16	45
Low	8	7	10	25
Family composition				
Single-parent	10	10	9	29
Stepparent	4	9	2	15
Original two-parent	16	9	22	47
Category (N)				
Aggressiveness	3	11	8	22
Hyperactivity	6	4	6	16
Social withdrawal	6	7	5	18
Attention control	15	6	13	34
X, Index of Severity				
Aggressiveness	4.73	5.14	4.70	
Hyperactivity	4.71	4.92	4.72	
Social withdrawal	5.87	5.49	4.77	
Attention control	5.71	5.16	5.57	
Total severity index	7.09	6.51	6.15	
Child's IQ (X) Ammons	115.3	114.3	120.0	

was underrepresented among children who received Information Feedback, whereas Hyperactivity and Poor Attention Control were overrepresented: Aggressiveness was overrepresented in the Parent Counseling group.

The fourth category in Table 1, Index of Severity, reflects the degree of reported behavioral disturbance for the children in each treatment group at the time of referral. This Mean Severity Index for each referral category represents the average score on that dimension for children in each of the different treatment groups. (The Mean Total Severity Index is the average score of the composite numbers developed for each child from the number of behavioral problems reported for him, the frequency of each report, and a weighting for degree of severity represented by each statement; see Appendix A, p. 234.) The three intervention groups did not differ significantly on this Total Index. However, the Information Feedback children received higher severity scores on Social Withdrawal and Attention Control than the other groups ($p<.05$).

Finally, there were no significant differences in Mean Ammons IQs for the children receiving the three types of treatments.

UTILIZATION OF SERVICES

Of a total of 152 referred families, 91 accepted and kept an initial interview. Of this number, 77 (85%) completed the treatment series offered. Sixty-four percent of the 91 families (58) came in for at least one follow-up interview.* Twenty-nine control families agreed to participate and completed their sessions. Twenty-five (86%) returned for at least one follow-up appointment.

Characteristics of clinicians in the different treatments (sex and level of experience) and the utilization of treatments (number of sessions, number of cases dropping out of treatment, and number of families coming in for at least one follow-up interview) are found in Table 2. There was no overlap among the staff providing the three types of service. For the purposes of this study, professional certification for independent private practice was the criterion of expert status for Child Therapy and Parent Counseling clinicians. Psychology and social work graduate students were considered to fall into the nonexpert category. For the Information Feedback group "expert" included only the two clinicians (Kaswan and Love) who had developed the approach. Other staff, as well as graduate students, were coached by them in the goals and techniques of an approach that in many ways runs counter to the traditional clinical stance of "giving help." For both years half of the

---

* Note, however, that follow-up grades were obtained for 80% of all cases.

Table 2. Formal Characteristics of Clinicians and Treatments

	Informaton Feedback (Ncases = 30)		Parent Counseling (Ncases = 28)		Child Therapy (Ncases = 33)	
	No. of Cases	%	No. of Cases	%	No. of Cases	%
Clinician						
Sex						
Male	23	76	7	25	8	24
Female	7	23	21	75	25	76
Experience Status						
Expert	20	67	21	75	31	94
Nonexpert	10	33	7	25	2	6
Treatments						
Total number clinic appointments	255		163		411	
X	8.5		5.8		12.4	
Missed and cancelled appointments	35	14	27	11	64	16
Cases in for follow-up	19	63	19	70	20	61
Cases discontinuing treatment	2	7	5	18	7	21

eight consultants would have qualified as "expert" on the usual professional-certification criterion. They were members of the Psychology Clinic staff; the other consultants were psychology graduate students. Only three consultants worked with cases during both years.

For each treatment group, a family was considered to have discontinued treatment before completion if less than one-half of the scheduled number of appointments for that intervention (and year) was made and kept. There were no instances in which clinicians advised early termination.

Comparison Between Treatment Groups

As shown in Table 2, in Information Feedback 30 families and teachers were involved in 255 appointments, with a mean of 8.5 and a range of 2–14 contacts per case. Two families came in for only two sessions and were considered to be terminators, providing a 7% dropout rate. Nineteen families (63%) returned for at least one follow-up session.

The mean number of clinic visits for Parent Counseling was 5.9, with a range of 1–13. Two cases were seen for an extended number of interviews, one for 12 sessions, another for 13, when counselors felt this necessary to tide parents over very difficult periods with their children. The mode for Parent Counseling was five sessions. Five families came in for only one or two interviews and so were considered terminators. This gave a dropout rate of 18%. Nineteen families (70%) came in for at least one follow-up session.

The mean number of meetings in the Child Therapy cases was 12.5, with a range of 1–20. Seven parents brought their children in for less than half the projected number of treatment sessions, and so were counted as having terminated prematurely, the therapist either not concurring or not being consulted in the decision to terminate. The dropout rate for Child Therapy was 21%. Twenty of the 33 families (61%) came in for at least one follow-up interview.

A check of Table 2 suggests that treatments were provided as planned. Approximately the expected number of appointments were made and kept for each type of intervention. A similar number of families from each group returned for follow-up sessions. The dropout rate was not related to length of treatment (Information Feedback = 7%, Parent Counseling = 18%, and Child Therapy = 21%), but these percentages represent small numbers of cases, and the overall dropout rate of 15% is low for a child guidance center population (Ross & Lacey, 1961).

Comparison Between the Two Years

Analysis of formal characteristics by year (Appendix B, Table 23) indicates that for Information Feedback and Parent Counseling there was no marked difference between Year I and II in the extent to which families remained in treatment. The lower number of contacts with Information Feedback and Child Therapy during Year II reflects the lower maximum number of sessions established for the second year. The dropout rate for Child Therapy differed for the two years in that all seven terminations occurred during the first year, none during the second. Missed and cancelled appointments, however, were higher for the second year (39) than for the first (29).

Differences in Treatment Utilization in Terms of SEL

Data reflecting the differential use of treatments by the three socioeconomic groups are summarized in Table 3. Middle socioeconomic level cases averaged fewer clinic appointments (7.9) than did Lo SEL (9.0) cases. Similarly, they dropped out of treatment at a slightly higher rate: 8 (18.2%) as compared to 2 (9.5%) for the Hi and 4 (15.4%) for Lo SEL. These figures probably reflect the unusual efforts in project planning to involve poorer families, for example, provision of transportation to campus. Even so, Lo

Table 3.   Clinic Appointments in Relation to Intervention Groups and Socioeconomic Level

	Information Feedback	Child Therapy	Parent Counseling	Total
Hi SEL	$n = 6$	$n = 7$	$n = 8$	$n = 21$
Total appts. kept	70	112	64	246
Mean no. of appts.	11.7	16	8	11.7
% Missed or cancelled	12.8	6.2	4.6	7.7
% Dropout	0	14.3	12.5	9.5
% Cases in for follow-up	83.3	71.4	62.5	67.0
% Appts. with father	65.7	26.8	34.4	39.8
Mid SEL	$n = 16$	$n = 16$	$n = 13$	$n = 45$
Total appts. kept	120	169	68	357
Mean no. of appts.	7.5	10.5	5.2	7.9
% Missed or cancelled	5.0	18.4	28.6	15.5
% Dropout	6.2	31.2	16.7	18.2
% Cases in for follow-up	62.5	62.5	76.9	67.0
% Appts. with father	49.2	25.9	52.4	39.1
Low SEL	$n = 8$	$n = 10$	$n = 7$	$n = 25$
Total appts. kept	65	130	31	226
Mean no. of appts.	8.1	13.0	4.4	9.0
% Missed or cancelled	30.8	22.3	17.1	23.9
% Dropout	12.5	10.0	25.0	15.4
% Cases in for follow-up	50.0	50.0	57.1	52.0
% Appts. with father	9.2	6.9	28.6	10.9
Total	$n = 30$	$n = 33$	$n = 28$	$n = 91$
Total appts. kept	255	411	163	829
Mean no. of appts.	8.5	12.5	5.9	9.1
% Missed or cancelled	13.7	16.2	10.5	15.5
% Dropout	6.7	21.2	17.8	15.4
% Cases in for follow-up	63.0	61.0	70.0	63.7
% Appts. with father	43.5	19.7	40.1	31.3

SEL families either missed or cancelled nearly a quarter as many appointments as they kept and only half of the group was available for follow-up interviews in the clinic. The difficulty of our Lo SEL groups in maintaining scheduled involvement in clinic treatment is in line with results reported by others (e.g., Speer et al., 1968; Baum et al., 1966).

Involvement of Fathers in the Three Groups

The importance of including fathers in treatment programs for children's behavior disorders has been emphasized periodically over the years (Towle, 1930; Lowrey, 1948; English, 1954; LeMasters, 1970). It has seldom been implemented in practice, however. For all families involved in this project, the one criterion for acceptance was that the entire family (everyone living in the home) should attend the first session in the clinic. It was emphasized that this included fathers or father surrogates in the home. Evening and Saturday appointments were set up whenever fathers' work schedules would have ruled out their attendance. In divorced families where one spouse was out of the home but lived in the local area both parents were requested to attend the initial interview. For continuing sessions, the involvement of the father was left up to the clinician. Information Feedback consultants emphasized the importance of fathers' presence at all sessions. Parent Counselors did too, according to case notes, though in a less uniform manner. There was much more variability in Child Therapists' recorded efforts to engage fathers in ongoing appointments.

Table 3 gives the percentage of father sessions in the clinic for each treatment group and each socioeconomic level. For Information Feedback, the higher the SEL the greater the number of father appointments, with Hi SEL fathers involved in 66%, Mid SEL 49%, and Lo SEL 9% of the clinic appointments for the case. For Child Therapy only a quarter of the appointments at both Hi and Mid SEL levels involved fathers, and Lo SEL fathers were present for only 7% of the appointments. In Parent Counseling 34% (Hi SEL), 39% (Mid SEL), and 29% (Lo SEL) appointments included fathers. For all socioeconomic levels combined, Information Feedback cases involved fathers in 44%, Parent Counseling in 40%, and Child Therapy in 20% of the family appointments. For all treatments combined, less than a third (31%) of all appointments included fathers.

The families of nonreferred children were seen for the same measures given to Information Feedback families. The nonreferred families had one or two feedback sessions and came in for follow-up sessions at the usual intervals. This group is not considered a treatment group because the families presumably were there to confirm rather than to change their behaviors. Their clinic sessions were conducted by a mature research psychologist with excellent interpersonal skills but no clinical orientation or training.* School personnel were not involved in project contacts with nonreferred families beyond the initial identification of the child and the provision of ratings by teachers. Of the original 29 control families, none dropped out of the initial series of contacts, and 25 (86%) returned to the clinic for at least one follow-up interview.

There are numerous sources of possible bias in conducting a study such as this. Secretaries who set up appointments and arranged follow-ups, project assistants who administered measures to clients, and other clinic staff neces-

* This was one of Bette Overman's many contributions to the project.

sarily knew the treatments to which families were assigned. Each worker was aware of the inherent hazards and tried to guard against differential attitudes and responses, but no one can estimate the effectiveness of such efforts. The comparable number of families in each treatment group who accepted followup appointments at least suggests that all families had generally similar reactions to the clinic staff and procedures.

The differential effects of the treatments as reflected in our outcome criteria are presented in the following chapter.

CHAPTER 8

Differential Outcomes
of Treatments

Outcomes for the three treatments are presented in terms of our most objective measures of pre- to posttreatment change: children's school grades and observers' ratings of children's behavior at school. The interrelationships between all outcome measures and the SEL of the family were explored, as were differences associated with the four types of problems demonstrated by the children.*

SCHOOL GRADES

Grades were obtained for the period from three semesters before treatment through at least the third semester following termination. This span included two or more follow-up intervals for almost all cases. Unless otherwise indicated, analyses reported below were based on the average of all grades which each child received at each grading period.

Pre- and Posttreatment Grades

Analyses of changes in grades over time for the three treatment groups indicated no overall differences in pre- and posttreatment grades between groups: a mixed-design, Group × Time analysis of variance yielded an F of 0.75. However there was a significant time effect ($F = 3.46$; $df = 3,192$; $p < .05$) and a Time × Group interaction ($F = 2.68$; $df = 6,192$; $p < .05$). The Time × Group interaction is shown graphically in Figure 9.†

---

* Portions of these data are also reported in Love, Kaswan, and Bugental, 1972. © 1972 by the American Psychological Association and reprinted by permission.

† Results are presented for 1-year intervals. A time trend analysis for one semester time intervals also yielded a significant Time × Group interaction ($F = 1.85$; $df = 12,385$; $p < .05$). One-year time intervals were employed because they give a clearer picture of changes.

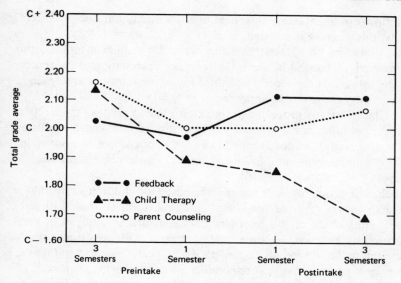

Figure 9. Pre- and posttreatment grades.

Figure 9 shows that there had been a general decline in grades for all three treatment groups during the 1-year period preceding referral for treatment. The average grade for referred children fell from 2.10† (three semesters before intake) to 1.89 (one semester before intake), a decline which is significant at near the .01 level ($t = 2.58$, $df = 1, 92$). Within the same period the grades of nonreferred children did not show any comparable decline. For these children, the average of their preintake grades was 2.62; the average of follow-up grades was 2.65. It seems unlikely, therefore, that the initial downward trend in the grades of referred children reflects more stringent grading policies in successively higher grades. Instead it seems to indicate the increasing deterioration in school performance that generally occurs when children are experiencing social and emotional problems. It should be noted that the 1 year preintake grades were assigned largely by teachers not involved in the identification of these children for referral for psychological help.

Figure 9 further shows that grade changes follow a different pattern for the three treatment groups from the time of intake. The decline in grades for children in Information Feedback appeared to be interrupted when treatment began; grade averages rose a fraction of a grade point by the time of

† 4 = A; 3 = B; 2 = C; 1 = D; 0 = F.

the first follow-up, maintaining this level over an additional two semesters. Statistically, this increase is not significant ($t = 1.32, df = 1, 92$).

Parent Counseling also interrupted the preintake decline in grades, but grades remained unchanged between the semester preceding and the semester following intake. At the second and third follow-up intervals a very slight improvement in grade averages appeared ($t = 0.50$).

For the Child Therapy group the preintake decline in grades (the steepest of the three curves, but not significantly so), continued uninterrupted during and following therapy. Grades dropped from 1.89 (one semester prior to intake) to 1.69 (three semesters following intake), a decrease significant at the .05 level ($t = 2.05; df = 1, 96$).*

Since behavior problems were the specific bases for children's referrals, a separate analysis was made of "conduct" grades since these should directly reflect the quality of the child's interpersonal behavior. An analysis of variance was used to compare the three treatment groups for two time periods (one semester preintake versus follow-up #3). *There was a trend* ($p < .10$) *for all groups to receive higher conduct grades following treatment* ($F = 3.10; df = 1, 64$). Improvement was slightly greater for Information Feedback but there was no significant difference between groups ($F = 1.97; df = 2, 64$), nor was there any interaction between group and time ($F = 1.9$).

Because of repeated findings in other aspects of the demonstration project which emphasize the importance of father-child interactions for these 8–12 year olds, we investigated the effect of father involvement on treatment outcomes. A Pearson r correlation was computed for the number of father appointments in the clinic with the difference in child's pre- and posttreatment grades. Although attempts had been made to include both parents in all two-parent families given Information Feedback or Parent Counseling, the father was often absent. Similar correlations with grade change were determined for mother appointments in single-parent families and for total number of appointments for each family. These analyses were done within each treatment group.

For Information Feedback families the correlation between father appointments and the child's grade improvement was $+.55$ ($p < .01$), for the 23 families with fathers. Since both other indices (number of mother appointments and total number of appointments for the cases) were not significantly associated with improved grades ($r = -.09$ and $+.35$, respective-

---

* The extent to which reported changes might be attributed to regression effects would seem to have been minimized by the fact that premeasures are based on time periods prior to referral. Thus regression effects should be the same for one semester preintake and one semester postintake. Survey of the data indicates that this effect seems possibly involved only for the Parent Counseling group.

ly), the father involvement seems of pivotal importance for the effectiveness of Information Feedback.

For Parent Counseling a very different pattern emerged. *Appointments involving the 22 fathers in this group were negatively* (though *not significantly*) correlated with pre-post improvement in grades ($r = -.26$).* On the other hand, for the six mother-as-only-parent families, the number of mother appointments was significantly associated with improved grades for Parent Counseling ($r = .60$, $p < .05$). For so small a number of cases, of course, this finding is only descriptively interesting. For this treatment group as a whole, the total number of appointments was negatively correlated with school improvement ($r = -.39$, $p < .05$). This would suggest that, except for mother-only families, the benefit accruing to parent counseled families occurs in the initial contacts; continuing the series may do more harm than good. The need for further investigation of length of counseling and possible differences between the responses of mothers and fathers to different treatment approaches seems evident.

For Child Therapy there was no significant relationship for any pattern of attendance at the clinic.

No reason is known for the negative relation between number of appointments for fathers and improvement in grades for the Parent Counseling group. It may be that one or two sessions are enough to identify problems and obtain recommendations. We speculate that contact continued beyond this phase may become very much like a form of brief therapy, a treatment which depressed grades according to our criteria. This similarity (between extended Parent Counseling series and Child Therapy which involves parents as well as children) is considered further in the next chapter.

In summary, the grades results indicate that Information Feedback and Parent Counseling stopped and slightly reversed the downward trend in the referred child's total grade averages (academic achievement and conduct). Child Therapy halted the decline in conduct grades but not in academic grades. For Information Feedback families, improved grades at school were positively related to the number of times the father came to the clinic, despite the low number of possible clinic sessions. The reverse was found for Parent Counseling, where higher frequencies of father visits were associated with declining grades in children.

For these referred children, interruption of progressive decline in school

---

* To examine whether these findings might be an artifact of SEL, we computed correlations between change in grades and the number of appointments with the father present for Hi and Mid SEL groups separately. (There were too few two-parent Lo SEL families to permit reliable correlations.) For Information Feedback, the r for Hi SEL was $+.57$; for Mid SEL $r = +.19$. For Parent Counseling, the r for Hi SEL was $-.40$; for Mid SEL $r = -.16$.

grades is evidence of improvement. The fact that the higher level of performance was maintained over time indicates that the improvement was probably not a chance finding. But it is disappointing that grades do not continue to advance to higher levels for either group. It may be that children's symptomatic difficulties decreased but psychological growth was not stimulated. We can only speculate as to whether some limitation in the two treatments is the basic factor involved or whether our outcome criterion is insensitive to further improvement. The critical role of teacher's expectations with respect to children's performance has been demonstrated amply (e.g., Rosenthal, 1966). Children's school records usually contain a description of their previous performance and it is possible that many teachers continue to expect the same level of achievement, whatever the child's current behavior. It may be recalled that in their adjective ratings teachers tended to differentiate with respect to children's negative qualities more often than to their more positive assets. Thus it seems possible that it is indeed difficult to overcome "negative halos."

Finally, it should be noted that we are reporting the *average* grades of two groups of children, each containing children representing a range of basic intellectual capacity and scholastic orientation. From this point of view, it may be unrealistic to expect means for the group to rise above the average grade for school children in general, the "C" to which grades had been restored by the two treatments. The question of individual fluctuations within the groups is explored in the next chapter.

Socioeconomic Level as Related to Changes in Grades

Figure 10 shows the differential outcomes for the three treatments in relation to the socioeconomic level of the families. *Although the overall SEL Group $\times$ Time interaction is only a trend ($F = 2.14$; $df = 4, 54$; $p < .10$), the slope for Information Feedback differs from that of the other two treatment methods: the higher the socioeconomic level of the family, the greater the increase in children's grades. Results for Parent Counseling suggest an opposite relationship. It seems to be most effective in improving grades of the lower socioeconomic group, only slightly less so for middle class, but falls off markedly in its effectiveness for the upper middle class families. Child Therapy did not lead to improvement in grades for any SEL group.*

If the analysis is limited to Information Feedback and Parent Counseling, the two treatments that interrupted the decline of grades, the interaction effect between social class, treatment group, and time is significant at better than the .05 level ($F = 4.01$; $df = 2, 36$).

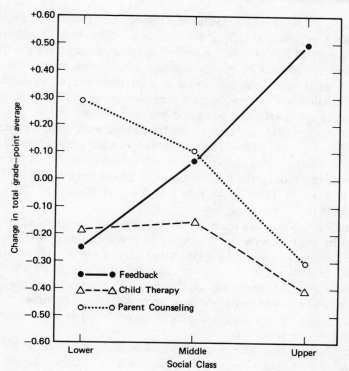

Figure 10. Differential outcomes for treatment groups in relation to socioeconomic level of the family.

Referral Categories as Related to Changes in Grades

Grade changes were examined for children with different types of referral problems to test the effectiveness of the various treatments. There were few interactions between referral categories and types of treatment, and only one that was significant: Information Feedback and Child Therapy (in that order) seem to have been relatively more effective for hyperactive children than was Parent Counseling ($F = 3.71$; $df = 2, 60$; $p < .05$). Since this is the only significant result, it may be due to chance.

Year I–Year II Comparison and Clinician Experience as Related to Changes in Grades

Grade changes were examined separately for Year I and Year II cases because of differences in treatment formats for the two years. Child Therapy, for example, was carried out exclusively by one professional therapist during the first year, whereas during the second, six different professional clinicians each carried two or three cases. In the Parent Counseling group, Year I cases were conducted by psychology and social work graduate students, whereas Year II cases were all carried by experienced social workers. Separate examination of each year's cases also provides a check on the possible infiltration of subtle selection or procedural changes over time.

Apparently the effects of each of the treatments were comparable for the two sets of cases seen during the two years. [Results were analyzed with a mixed-design Group × Time (intake versus third follow-up) × Year analysis of variance. No significant differences or trends were found for year ($F = 0.01$), Year × Time ($F = 0.09$) or Year × Group × Time ($F = 0.11$) effects.]

A separate analysis was made of the Information Feedback cases carried primarily by the two consultants who developed the approach, Kaswan and Love, in comparison with other consultants in this intervention. Although their cases initially (at first follow-up) had shown greater improvement than other feedback cases, there was no difference in the improvement of cases carried by these two presumably most committed consultants as compared to the cases seen by the other consultants ($F = 0.16$) in the amount of total grade improvement.

Grade changes thus were not influenced by differences in the number of therapists carrying child cases, the experience level of parent counselors, or the commitment of the consultants in the Information Feedback approach. Nor did the greater number of treatment sessions in the first-year therapy and feedback interventions yield more change than the shorter second-year formats.

The finding that differences in treatment outcomes were unrelated to level of clinician's experience aligns our findings with those who have reported similar results, for example, Wallach and Strupp (1964) and McNair and Lorr (1964). However, as Cartwright and Vogel (1960), among others, have noted, there are settings and conditions where successful treatment is related closely to the clinician's experience. We suspect that the latter would hold mainly where experience is related closely to complex rules of inference which must be learned by both clinician and patient. In the more behaviorally or situationally oriented interventions, however, like our parent counseling, amount of clinician's experience is presumably of less importance.

Discussion of School Grade Results

Two findings are of particular interest.

The failure of Child Therapy to interrupt the pattern of deteriorating school performance for any group of children in this sample was surprising. We had expected that this treatment might not work well with lower socio-economic families in which it might be difficult for parents to bring their children for a 12 or 20 week treatment series; parental concerns in these families, moreover, might be geared to more immediate practical problems (Sager et al., 1968) than to the psychodynamic mechanisms considered important by therapists. Among the middle- and upper-class families in our study, however, psychotherapy was accepted widely and generally considered the treatment of choice for a wide range of problems of all ages. This unexpected negative finding is discussed at the end of the chapter, in the context of all the outcome comparisons.

Information Feedback worked better for Hi SEL families; Parent Counseling worked better for Lo. We were aware of Becker's (1962) conclusion that "working class families focus more on conformity to external proscriptions (as in their occupational roles) while middle class parental values center more on self-direction" (p. 171). We had also noted Frank's (1961) earlier comments that lower-class families respond more favorably to suggestion and advice from expert sources than do upper-middle-class families, that well-educated people deal most comfortably in situations in which their insights and verbal skills are employed, and that for them directive methods are less desirable. But we had not anticipated that these differences would emerge in so clear-cut a fashion. Several hypotheses are considered which may account for the relation between the two effective treatments and SEL.

PARENTAL SEX DIFFERENCES IN RESPONSE TO THE TREATMENTS

The correlations between grade improvement and father involvement in treatment show that fathers responded best to Information Feedback, least to Parent Counseling. The mothers' differential response to the three treatments is less clear, but the data indicate a possibility that mothers who are single parents may respond best to the more directive Parent Counseling. We suspect that there may be a real difference in mothers' and fathers' responses, though this is hard to separate from the difference in Hi and Lo SEL reactions to the two effective interventions. There is evidence that working-class mothers tend to be susceptible to expert opinion with respect to child rearing (e.g., Hoffman, 1960). Since the Lo SEL group contained a high percentage of mother-only families, the generally greater responsiveness of this group to the Parent Counseling approach may be due largely to the Lo SEL mothers' responsiveness to directive counseling. On the other hand, the relatively nondirective, cognitive approach of Information Feedback might well have more appeal for fathers, especially the economically more successful ones who would be likely to respond well to a problem-solving approach. There was a general impression among project personnel that fathers at all SELs tended to have a more immediate and stronger positive response to the initial description of the Information Feedback approach than did mothers. Our anecdotal impression also indicated that fathers were often the ones who made both the first and greatest changes in response to the feedback materials.

In a more general sense, these results may reflect parental feelings of autonomy and power versus dependency and helplessness. It would seem that, in general, the idea of "being told" something about oneself or being given advice by an expert has both a positive and a negative effect. The positive value lies in the hope that we can depend on sources and resources outside ourselves for help and understanding when we cannot cope on our own. The opposite reaction may stem from the resistance to external control that seems to coexist with dependency or solution seeking behavior. Brehm (1966) and his co-workers have elaborated one aspect of this counterreaction to external influence which they term "reactance": the desire to feel oneself a free agent and to reinstate the concept of having a free choice whenever limitations on behavior are threatened or implied. From this perspective, our Socioeconomic Level × Type of Treatment interactions seem to reflect a preference for free choice to do whatever one feels is best, to the degree to which the individual parent perceives himself as competent to proceed alone. In our sample the relatively successful Hi SEL father, for all his difficulties in his parental role, is in a very different position from the divorced Lo SEL mother who has few personal or environmental supports to draw upon. The Hi SEL father may place high value on his autonomy, whereas the relief of being able to rely on outside help may have much appeal for the Lo SEL mother. This speculation would be consistent with the family measure findings discussed in the preceding section. It is related as well to the reactions of the individual within the family group, particularly to emerging needs for autonomy as the child develops. It also seems important to consider as we assess the reactions of aggressive and hyperactive children who seem to experience difficulty in adapting to the confines and restrictions of the classroom situation.

COGNITIVE COMPLEXITY AND VERBAL SOPHISTICATION

Our outcome pattern may also be related to differences in verbal sophistication and in familiarity with the type of cognitively complex tasks involved in Information Feedback. Our relatively verbal Hi SEL group can be assumed to be attracted to situations that place heavy demands on attention. In contrast, our Lo SEL group, which had difficulties in our verbal communication tasks (Ammons FRPV, Communication Task), may respond more to situations that demand less sophisticated verbal performance and less attention to complex cognitive manipulations. Information Feedback unquestionably poses a more intricate situation than Parent Counseling. In the former intervention, parents must attend to and integrate a diversity of verbal and visual stimuli. They are given information from family ratings, teacher ratings, parent and teacher questionnaires, etc., and are asked to compare and analyze this material for themselves. Since the Hi SEL parents were verbally sophisticated and used to complex cognitive situations, they were in the best position to take full advantage of these techniques which demanded concentrated attention. In the Parent Counseling intervention, parents were required only to describe the situation in their own way, respond to direct questions, and accept the suggestions of a counselor.

From a specific theoretical point of view, the observed interaction between socioeconomic status and the effectiveness of different interventions may be related to McGuire's mediational principle of attitude change (1969). According to this principle, attitude change derives as a combined function of attention and yielding. Intelligence is positively related to attention but negatively related to yielding. Correspondingly, high intelligence groups (our upper-middle group) are relatively more influenceable in complex situations which place heavy demands on attentional components; low intelligence* groups (our lower-class group) are relatively more influenceable in simple situations which are easily understood and require only simple conformity.

In further research we are planning to reduce the complexity of the feedback procedures, particularly by simplifying the paper and pencil tasks. These simplifications should provide more exact information about the differential role of verbal sophistication and cognitive complexity for the different SEL groups.

DIFFERENCES BETWEEN PROFESSIONS PROVIDING TREATMENT

Another possible reason for the relation between Information Feedback, Parent Counseling, and socioeconomic status may lie in differences in the orientation and experience of the two professions providing the two services. Parent Counseling was conducted either by social workers or by graduate students under social work supervision. Information Feedback was carried out by psychology staff and graduate students. It is probable that the social workers as a group had had more direct previous experience with families from lower socioeconomic levels than the psychologists. Since it is generally assumed that clinicians are most effective if they are familiar with the sociocultural characteristics of their client, it would seem reasonable that the traditional experience of social workers would give them a generalized advan-

---

* Intelligence is here defined only in a purely operational sense. We make no inferences with respect to the relation of these IQ scores to any "basic" intellectual capacity, however conceived.

tage in their dealings with persons at lower socioeconomic levels. (This difference, if it indeed obtained, is being lessened rapidly by recent developments within psychology.) Similarly, the more detached, ostensibly nondirective stance of the psychologists who elaborated the Information Feedback approach might well reflect their middle-class orientation toward autonomy, and hence imply an affinity between themselves and clients with similar predilections. The reader will recall that a major purpose in the development of the approach had been to facilitate adult reliance on their own resources for change.

INTERPERSONAL EFFECTIVENESS OF LO SEL CHILDREN

A final factor which may have contributed to the results may have been the relatively greater interpersonal effectiveness of many Lo SEL as compared to higher SEL children. As noted in Chapter 5, many Lo SEL children were referred largely because of their aggressive behavior in relation to adults. Both mothers and teachers saw them as quite effective in relation to peers. It may be speculated, therefore, that relatively slight changes in the parents could be enough to enable these children to adjust their behaviors, to become more acceptable to adults. Mid and Hi SEL children, especially those at Hi SEL levels, usually had serious problems of interpersonal effectiveness with both adults and peers. For these children, more extensive alterations in adult behaviors may have been required. This is, again, entirely speculative.

In summary, the grades data indicate that successful intervention for children's adjustment problems occurred when the parents were the predominant focus of treatment. Psychotherapy which focused on the psychological state of the child did not result in improved grades. Analysis of interaction between family SEL and the three treatment groups indicates that a cognitive self-help approach like Information Feedback is more effective for higher SEL families, especially for fathers, whereas direct counseling is better utilized by lower SEL parents, perhaps especially mothers. It is interesting to note that in both effective interventions the goal is to get new information to the parents about their child.

Grades changes within any treatment were not differentially related to the type of problem the child showed, whether it consisted of predominantly aggressive, hyperactive, inhibited, or distractible behavior. The critical choice, therefore, appears to be the matching of the treatment to the characteristics of the available parent(s), (e.g., SEL and perhaps sex).

SCHOOL OBSERVERS' RATINGS

The second major criterion for comparing the outcomes of the three treatments was change in observers' ratings of the child's behavior in the school setting. The procedures for obtaining these classroom and playground ratings are described in Chapter 5. Changes were anticipated only for those situations in which substantial initial differences had been found between referred and nonreferred children. Our analysis of adjective ratings was made in terms of two factors, the Negative Social Impact and the Positive Social Impact of the rated behavior (see Appendix A, pp. 237–242). For the observers' ratings of the child's behavior at school only the social negativity factor showed significant referred/nonreferred differences in all three situations (playground, child to teacher in classroom, and child to peers in the classroom) for both years (see Chapter 5). For the positive factor, referred/nonreferred differences were not consistently significant. In addition, there was a marked difference for this factor in the ratings of Year I versus Year II. Factor II results, therefore, are not reported here.*

Time trends were studied for the entire project period, from original (referral) ratings through both the second and third follow-up intervals. A mixed-design analysis of variance was used to analyze time trends for Negative Social Impact for the three treatment groups in each of the three rating situations. Results were statistically significant only for ratings of children made on the playground. Apparently, limitations on children's behavior in the classroom decreased the likelihood of variability that otherwise could be obtained in behavioral ratings such as these. *On the playground, however, all three treatment groups showed an overall decrease in ratings of social negativity made at the second follow-up period relative to ratings made at the time of referral* ($F_{Time} = 15.66$; $df = 1, 57$; $p < .01$). In this analysis, there were no differences between treatment groups ($F_{Group} = 1.87$; $df = 2, 57$). The Group × Time interaction was also nonsignificant ($F = .58$; $df = 2, 57$). However, the pattern of pre-post change was consistent: slightly larger for Feedback, intermediate for Parent Counseling, and least for Child Therapy. The results are shown in Figure 11.

The findings at the third follow-up were essentially the same as those shown in Figure 11, although the number of cases by the third follow-up

---

* This year effect resulted from a change in the method of selection of the random children. Chapter 5 describes the fact that, for methodological reasons, ratings of referred and nonreferred children were always compared with the ratings given random children for an equivalent time period. During Year I "random" children were chosen from "visible" children in the rating situation. Analysis of ratings at the end of the first year revealed that this practice resulted in the identification of highly active children as randoms. This had the effect of skewing C scores for factor II, in which activity was a major component. To correct for this, randoms during the second year were chosen from school lists. Consequently, there is a clear difference between Years I and II on this factor. Since teacher ratings of the referred and nonreferred children on factor II indicate no difference between Year I and Year II *children,* we conclude, therefore, the two groups cannot be considered comparable.

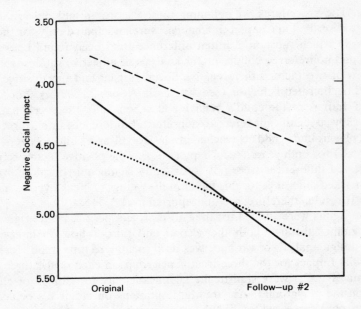

Figure 11. Decrease in ratings of Negative Social Impact made by school observers for children's playground behavior, pre- and posttreatment.

(about two years after intake) was sharply reduced to six cases for Information Feedback and seven for each of the other two treatment groups. It was obviously easier to get grades for children from their new schools than it was to obtain additional behavioral observations in the new settings. Therefore we had many fewer children for whom we had third follow-up behavior ratings than was true for follow-up grades.

The results in Figure 11 show that *all* children appear less socially negative in their playground behavior, a change which was temporally related to their experience in the clinic. This finding parallels the comparable improvement in conduct grades found for children in all three treatment groups. The school observation data yielded no significant finding for socioeconomic level or referral category.

A number of supplementary indications of change were contained in teacher ratings. Since some of these indices are subject to bias and the results are often based on relatively small numbers of cases, they are reported in Appendix B, Table 24. We may note here, however, that the supplementary findings confirmed the grade results in showing greatest improvement for Information Feedback, and least improvement for Therapy.

SUMMARY AND DISCUSSION

Our data clearly indicate that for grade-school adjustment problems, interventions focusing on parents result in more improvement in the child's school behavior than does time limited psychotherapeutic treatment for the child. The lesser effectiveness of Child Therapy was consistent at all socioeconomic levels.

It is possible that for child psychotherapy to have sufficient impact on school grades, a longer or more intensive treatment series is required. In some studies, such as that of Maas et al. (1955), the successful outcome of child psychotherapy is directly related to length of treatment. Levitt has conjectured, on the basis of the Maas study and his own investigations of the characteristics of defectors from child therapy, that "improvement is a function of at least 40 treatment interviews; a lesser number actually makes the patient worse" (1960, p. 90). Even if this time requirement should be valid, however, it markedly limits the population that will benefit because of the restrictions inherent in the time, money, and motivation necessary for such sustained treatment, especially in the absence of intermediate signs of improvement and with the demonstration of other, more direct and efficient methods of intervention.

Heinecke and Goldman (1960) concluded from their survey of child therapy research that treatment provided beneficial results but that for a significant number of cases the improvement occurred after the close of therapy. Our data would not support such a conclusion, unless a longer time interval than a year were posited before improvement should be expected to appear.

A second possibility remains open: that the child given psychotherapy may have benefited in ways not reflected in our criteria. It is easy to question the appropriateness of the choice of grades as criteria. Though they were chosen because of their relative objectivity, and do represent a socially accepted index of performance and adaptive effectiveness, a more humanistic orientation may hold that grades simply represent a measure of conformity. Many therapists take such a position. In doing so, however, they must recognize that they are representing a different value system than that held by most parents and teachers. Indeed, this added source of adult incongruity may set up an additional complexity for the child.

A question can be raised as to the extent to which the seven therapists who treated the 33 clients are representative of nonmedical child therapists in general. Kiesler (1967) has warned against the assumption of uniformity of treatments just because an experimental design provides a label, and this may play some unknown part in our results. Our professional clinicians were selected to be representative of psychologists and social workers who worked as child therapists in both agency and private practice settings. At the time, they described themselves as identified with the definition of child therapy that we had outlined. Within our group of therapists, the fact that there was no significant difference in outcome of Year I therapy cases (all carried by one clinician) and Year II cases (conducted by six clinicians) would suggest that therapist variability was not a strongly operative factor. A clearer description of how these therapists utilized the clinical hours is provided in the case illustrations in the next chapter.

An additional possibility to be considered is that the group means are misleading and that individual cases might reflect strikingly different outcomes than the means suggest (Shapiro, 1968). For our population, however, only three of the 33 children receiving child therapy showed a rise of half a grade point after therapy. Of these three, only one demonstrated this improvement consistently over the follow-up interval. For the other two, there was equal variability in a negative direction over one or more follow-up periods. Furthermore, of these three children, two were treatment dropouts, their therapy having been discontinued by their parents before one-half the available series had taken place. Therefore, for this sample, group trends reflecting no improvement are not contradicted by individual instances of success.

The fact that therapy, like the other two interventions, is followed by some improvement in conduct grades and in ratings of the child's behavior on the playground may reflect a general tendency for children's behavior to improve somewhat whenever they receive any special attention. The relative weakness of the effect for Child Therapy, however, indicates that the essential attention comes from adults important in the life situation and that this cannot be replaced quickly by a relationship with a therapist in a clinic. The general conclusion seems to be that when significant adults focus on a child's difficulty and try to ameliorate the context within which he lives, improvement results. When the responsibility for adaptive improvement is placed directly on the child, there is little or no progress in terms of our criteria. Thomas, Chess, and Birch (1968, p. 177) report a similar high correlation between parents' positive reaction to parent guidance and child's concurrent improvement. Brookover et al. (1968) report failure of direct counseling of the child to bring about significant change in either a child's self-concept or his school achievement. They suggest that the best way to effect these goals is through work with parents: "Working through an already established significant other is more likely to be effective than developing a new significant other" (p. 506). Also, the child generally has little direct power to change the situation or to influence others apart from resistance and indirect manipulation. Parents and teachers, on the other hand, obviously exercise primary control over the child's physical and interpersonal environment at this age level.

Finally, in the comparison between Information Feedback and Parent Counseling, there is a small but consistent tendency in most measures for Feedback to demonstrate a wider range and a higher level of improvement. This may represent only the appeal of a new approach; perhaps the use of the videotapes was initially intriguing. These questions are currently being studied through our process measures. On the basis of relevance to our outcome criteria, however, it seems that one probable factor in the favorable results for Information Feedback was the inclusion of school personnel in the feedback process. This was seen as accomplishing two things: (1) increasing the teacher's awareness of the child's objective behavior and the teacher's role in relation to the child; and (2) facilitating communication between home and school. Both should contribute to some reduction in incongruous expectations and demands set up for the child in the two situations. The outcomes were not, however, attributable to a halo effect of teachers' participation in the project; no children were receiving grades or ratings from the same teachers at the outset of treatment and at follow-up intervals.

From a methodological perspective, these results show the value of (1) using multiple outcome measures, (2) including both parents in clinical interventions, and (3) drawing cases from a socioeconomically heterogeneous sample. Congruent results from the different outcome measures, obtained by different persons from different perspectives, add to the confidence attributable to these results. Inclusion of both parents, where available, yielded results that are consonant with those reported in the family comparisons, where the father's role was seen as pivotal in the distinction between referred and nonreferred groups. If only the mother had been included in the treatments, as is often the case in child psychotherapy research, no relation between improvement and parental functioning would have been apparent. Finally, it is clear that use of a socioeconomically homogeneous sample, such as an upper-middle- or lower-class group, would have led to very different conclusions about the effectiveness of the treatments. If only an upper-middle-class sample had been used, the results in favor of the feedback approach, would have been very striking, as Figure 11 demonstrates. If only a Lo SEL group had been used, then the Parent Counseling approach would clearly have been revealed as most effective. The interaction obtained between type of treatment and socioeconomic level will permit a testing of alternative explanations in future studies.

CHAPTER 9

Successful and Unsuccessful Cases in Each Treatment

The case material in this chapter was chosen to complement the quantitative data presented in the preceding chapter with a qualitative picture of the treatment interactions. Since any psychological intervention can fail to be helpful, or may even appear to make things worse in individual instances (e.g., Rogers, 1967; Betz, 1963), we identified the six children in each treatment group with the most extreme grade changes, that is, the three with the most improved grades and the three whose grades declined most. We reviewed the case folders for all 18 children and selected the records that seemed most illustrative of the three treatment processes for inclusion here. For Information Feedback and Parent Counseling, two cases showing improvement in grades and one showing a posttreatment decrease in grades were selected. These cases seemed to offer sufficient illustrative material to represent important features of the process and effect of each intervention. For Child Therapy, we chose two cases that showed the most improved grades for this group and three cases whose grades decreased substantially after treatment.

The grade changes for these children are presented in Table 1. A one point change represents one letter grade: for example, $+1.00$ = B to A, -1.00 = loss of one grade level, for example, C to D. The change in observers' ratings on the playground is recorded whenever both pre and post data were available. (Names and some details have been altered to prevent identification of children or families.)

Table 1. Changes in Grade Averages of Most and Least Improved Cases in each Treatment Group

Information Feedback	$+1.19$	$+1.07$	$+1.06$	$-.56$	$-.62$	$-.81$
Parent Counseling	$+1.01^a$	$+1.00$	$+.63$	$-.44$	$-.87$	-1.06
Child Therapy	$+.75^a$	$+.69$	$+.50^a$	$-.87$	-1.25	-1.25

^{a} Identifies children who were treatment dropouts.

INFORMATION FEEDBACK

Case 1: Grade Change, +1.19; Playground Rating Change, +3.75

A 10½ year old boy, the younger of two sons of a Mid SEL, intact family, Roy was in Referral Category III, Social Withdrawal, with a high degree of severity.

SCHOOL REFERRAL DATA

"Doesn't concentrate, not motivated; bothers other children; pulls out and eats his hairs and eyebrows; many nervous habits, can't keep hands off other children, restless; does little work; practically a non-reader; craves attention." Binet IQ, 107; all academic grades D or F; F in effort and work habits; D in citizenship; attendance very good. Parents' initial response to school referral: mother interested, father suspicious but willing to try if evening hours available.

FAMILY

Father's occupation was given as cook; his chief interest, his union activities. The mother, aged 30, was employed as a bank teller. The family owned their three-bedroom home in a middle-class neighborhood.

TREATMENT FORMAT

Male consultant, experienced. There were nine appointments, none missed or cancelled, seven involving the father; there was one follow-up session. Excerpts from intervention notes indicated that there were two feedback sessions with parents and child, three with parents alone. One example of the materials used in feedback came from the low accuracy scores on the Family Communication Task: father and son both failed to make correct choices based on the other's descriptions. Family members made their own inferences about how father and son communicated, and questioned whether these two generally paid very close attention to each other.

In another session, profiles of individual family member's ratings of excerpts from televised family interactions were shown. The family noted that while there was generally good agreement among the three of them about their interactions (e.g., how angry one was with respect to another), the mother rated the child's behavior as controlling while the father considered the same behavior as rude. In yet another appointment the parents paid considerable attention to analyses of their Behavior Inventories as they went through their responses in some detail with the consultant. They made few comments except while covering the section of the inventory which described the affectional behaviors of parents in relation to the child. After looking at their own responses to these items, the mother said that it looked as though they were not showing Roy any affection. The father agreed and they talked at some length about this.

The teacher and counselor in their one session at the clinic viewed parts of the family videotape and studied profiles of the adjective ratings made by teacher and child of themselves, each other, and how each expected to be rated by the other. The parents and the consultant met once with the principal and teacher at the school. In this session, the parents emphasized that they considered the child's difficulties at school as largely the school's problem. In his turn the teacher enumerated both his concern for and frustration with Roy. He felt that Roy "hungered" for affection, but that as the teacher he could not give him the individual attention he craved. The parents agreed to work with the teacher but continued to insist on the school's primary responsibility for the child's behavior while there.

At a follow-up interview 6 months after termination, there was little verbal discussion of family changes or of the earlier clinic experience. The stress of the public nature of the family room (in which most Information Feedback sessions were conducted) was increased markedly. The father appeared particularly angry and resistant to the observers and consultant, though he made no verbal complaint. The family presented a united front, attending to each other to the exclusion of the project workers. They did not verbalize any recognition of improvement (though the schoolteacher's and observers' ratings definitely did). The father and son seemed to have greatly increased their verbal and eye contact. The boy especially appeared more spontaneous and self-reliant. He was the most outspoken of the three, in marked contrast to his former quite inhibited behavior.

Case 2: Grade Change, +1.06

This 11 year old boy had been adopted as an infant by his Hi SEL mother during a previous marriage; her current (second) marriage was of 3 years' duration. The referred child was the mother's only child; the stepfather had a grown family from his previous marriage. Referral Category: Attention Control, moderate severity.

SCHOOL REFERRAL DATA

Easily distracted, restless; poor self-control; argumentative.

FAMILY

The mother, aged 40, was a very nervous, uncertain person who often lost her temper. She felt her husband was jealous of the stepson, Tim. The stepfather, 53, was reported to be very rough (physically and psychologically) with both mother and son. He stated that use of his strength and authority had worked out well with his first family and was therefore appropriate for Tim. He had 2 years of college and was a successful (but exceptionally hard working) engineer. He refused to state his salary but the home and location implied a very high income.

TREATMENT FORMAT

Male consultant, inexperienced. Twelve appointments were kept (two with school personnel), six missed or cancelled; nine appointments involved the father; there was one follow-up session. This was the only Information Feedback case that utilized this many sessions. The father was very difficult to involve in the tasks, obviously fighting them by his lateness, cancellations, and argumentative discussions; but he continued to accept appointments and to show up for most of them. He tended always to want to debate and refute the feedback materials and did not enter into many discussions of the data with the family.

FOLLOW-UP

The videotaped interaction showed more attention directed toward the boy by the father: more looking at him, more verbalization directed to him; once he gave him a conspiratorial wink. The father also smiled at both wife and child and was more courteous and thoughtful in his behavior. In contrast to his adamant silence throughout much of the first tape, he responded to every remark made to him. There was generally less tension and hostility expressed among the family triad, both verbally and nonverbally, in the follow-up tape. As with the first case described, however, increase of interaction within the family was accompanied by a very strong assertion of exclusion of the consultant, camera, and possible observers. This father explicitly and adamantly refused to participate in the repetition of any of the original tasks beyond the problem definition. Yet he (personally) had accepted the follow-up appointment without hesitation.

Our speculation was that this father (who had previously used his extremely busy schedule as an excuse to break appointments) had in fact welcomed and utilized a chance to reenact the part of the first session that he had reluctantly observed in viewing the videotape. In "his" version, the follow-up, he was much pleasanter with his family and much more powerful and dominant with respect to the project staff. He softened his stand on the one hand, and toughened it on the other. It should be clear that this father remained a very gruff and critical man. In the interval since the school meetings, he had again become critical of the child's behavior, though not to the same extreme, according to the mother. We are describing a tempering, rather than removal, of the original negative behaviors. In addition, he showed interest and attention to the child, behaviors which had been conspicuously absent in the original tape. The mother and son seemed more relaxed and not at all surprised by the father's different behavior during the follow-up session. Their reaction was our only direct evidence that the father's behavior change was not just assumed for this occasion.

Case 3: Grade Change, −0.81

This 8 year old Caucasian girl was fourth in a family of five children, all girls except for the youngest; both natural parents were in the home, plus a 12 year old boy vaguely referred to as a relative. The maternal grandmother was also present, staying with the family on a protracted visit. The home was a rented three-bedroom house in a lower-middle-class area; the income was quite marginal for a family of seven. Referral Category: Attention Control, high degree of severity.

SCHOOL REFERRAL DATA

"Poor and extremely slow learner; will not try; gives up; no amount of encouragement or praise is successful in getting her to try; lack of attention or interest."

FAMILY

Father (30), a technical illustrator, high school graduate, was unsure of desire to participate at the clinic; the mother (30), also a high school graduate, was initially favorable to the idea of coming to the clinic though she did not consider that the child had any serious problems. Mother, target child, and one female sibling were all extremely obese.

TREATMENT FORMAT

Female consultant, expert. There were four sessions in Information Feedback format in which content was covered very slowly; the family pace would indeed be termed lethargic. The parents were polite and fairly affable. There was less concern and constraint about observation than in almost any family. Each appointment seemed a pleasant, innocuous family outing. After four sessions, illness of the consultant caused a 7 week interruption; meanwhile the mother-in-law, still visiting in the home, broke her hip, occasioning an additional delay. During this interim, the schoolteacher and principal became increasingly concerned about the child's bizarre, isolated behavior and requested psychological testing. This was finally done by the consultant in the child's home as a semiemergency measure. (The mother did not drive, the father could not get off from work, etc.) Standard psychological test results indicated an exceedingly disturbed, withdrawing child with very poor reality testing, very primitive and undifferentiated conceptual patterns, and much concern about her obesity. Her distress over her weight was relayed to the mother, along with information as to how thorough physical and endocrinological examination could be obtained at no cost. The consultant visited the school several times and conferred with teachers as the child's behavior was visibly deteriorating. The mother was invited to each of these school conferences by the principal. The principal reported that the mother seemed annoyed because the daughter talked a great deal about the consultant and often expressed a desire to see her. The mother also reported being disturbed by the child's interest in playing with a neighborhood boy, but did not seem concerned about her school behavior. She agreed to attend the final school appointment, though she declined for her husband who could not leave his work. And she herself did not appear when the time came.

FOLLOW-UP

The family came in for one follow-up but were bland and nonresponsive to materials (except the videotapes, which they chuckled at and seemed to enjoy). The parents had not followed through on the referral for physical examination for the daughter. They felt she was doing all right and were more concerned about their many financial and family worries at this time. They were also considering moving. The child's behavior in this situation was not nearly so bizarre as it had appeared at school. She was, however, completely nonresponsive (especially with the consultant). This was in marked contrast to the evident pleasure she had manifested in the interactions during previous clinic, home, and school contacts.

It was felt by project members that the more personal and active role taken by the consultant because of the seriousness of the child's withdrawing behavior had been incompatible with the methods and goals of Information Feedback and had been disruptive in this context: the relationship had become very important to the child and had simultaneously provoked an angry (possibly jealous) response in the mother, obliterating the minimal recognition she seemed to have about her daughter's isolated, socially withdrawn state.

Information Feedback Summary

In the two improved cases the father apparently manifested most behavioral change within the family, though each did so in quite idiosyncratic ways. The father in the final (unimproved) case was a passive, pale man who hardly showed up in the heavily feminine environment and who appeared untouched by the feedback experience. The fathers in the "successful" cases appeared to show increased involvement in familial interactions and their negativity seemed redirected toward the source of external stress (the clinic). We are checking to determine whether, in fact, a father's active aggression against a clear source of discomfort for all the members of his family (the observers, the recording equipment) might not in fact receive positive evaluative ratings if seen as his coming to an active defense of himself and his family. If so, a tentative correlation (change in father's positive and active involvement accompanied by a decrease in the child's immature and anxious behavior) might be evidenced here. It can only be checked for Information Feedback families since neither of the other two groups viewed their videotapes or saw observers' ratings. The hypothesis is that given an opportunity to evaluate via the videotape what actually occurred in the family in the observed situation, fathers were (as a group) surprised by the strength they showed. They then seemed to apportion and direct this strength more in accord with the way they would like to behave. Mothers and children by and large seemed to support the father's new manner of assumption of the responsible protective role. Some pilot data that provide tentative support for this concept are presented in the next chapter.

PARENT COUNSELING

Case 1: Grade Change, + 1.01; Playground Rating Change, + 1.12

Mike, a 10 year old, was the only child of a middle-class divorced mother who remarried between time of school referral and the intake appointment in the clinic. Referral Category: Aggressiveness, moderate severity.

SCHOOL REFERRAL DATA

"Due to his lack of self-control, he seldom completes any assignment and is working on a lowered grade level. Very belligerent. Has no respect for authority, is a continual nuisance. Lacks pride. Talks a lot. Seeks attention."

FAMILY

The new stepfather was a cameraman; the natural father owned a restaurant in another state and maintained no contact with his son; the mother was a beautician. In the initial interview she stated that she had had to work all her life and now with her new marriage had her first opportunity to stay at home; she looked forward to this greatly.

TREATMENT FORMAT

Female counselor; nonexpert. There was only the initial clinic appointment; additional contacts were politely but firmly refused by the parents after the intake interview. They stated that they felt the presence of the new father in the home and the opportunity for the mother to stay home would take care of the problem. Outcome results suggest that the parents were right; the intake staff, on the other hand, felt strongly that the parents were superficial, selfish, and resistant in their attitude, as they felt this boy was very inhibited and emotionally deprived. The grade pattern indicates an immediate decline following the marriage (follow-up #1) but increasing improvement thereafter. The family declined to accept a follow-up appointment.

Case 2: Grade Change, + 0.63; Playground Rating Change, + 1.75

The referred child was Carl, a 9 year old boy, from an intact, black, Lo SEL family who owned their three-bedroom house. Referral Category: Aggressiveness, moderate severity.

SCHOOL REFERRAL DATA

"Restless, hyperactive behavior, frequent clowning; unable to control temper; continually fighting, sudden outbursts of anger."

FAMILY

In the initial interview the parents indicated they had three sons, with the referred child, Carl, being the youngest. During clinic sessions, it later came out that there were 11 people living in the home. The family composition was never entirely clear. The father, 51, was a maintenance man; the mother, 43, did babysitting. The school had contacted the mother several times during the semester and requested her to come to school to talk about Carl's difficulties but she had not responded. When called again by the principal to ask permission to refer Carl to the clinic, the mother had acquiesced without comment.

TREATMENT FORMAT

Female counselor, expert. The family was seen for three conjoint interviews by an experienced social worker; Carl had one diagnostic play session and a battery of psychological tests was administered by a psychology graduate student. The family came in for two follow-up appointments.

Parents were seen as a fairly intelligent, excessively polite couple with the mother appearing "overwhelmingly dominating in both physical size and manner."* In the interview the parents revealed that Carl was enuretic and had many additional problems. They were afraid that he had suffered brain injury at birth. They responded well to hearing test results which emphasized that while he was developing slowly, he was not retarded and did have the ability to learn. Family patterns which encouraged his childishness and irresponsibility were discussed and alternative behaviors outlined which would provide external controls and encourage his own growth. The role of the father as an important model for the child was stressed.

FOLLOW-UP

At 6 months the clinician reported Carl's behavior as much more age-appropriate than when previously seen, and he was apparently much more verbal. Both parents seemed reassured and more approving of him. However, concerns over homework continued and the father remained notably passive and submissive to the mother.

At the 1 year follow-up, the family was much less satisfied with Carl and with their total family situation than they had been 6 months previously. Much of the boy's restlessness, distractibility, and immaturity were still apparent and seemed less acceptable and more irritating to the parents than ever. The clinical impression was that they were less worried about his basic capacity and so were critical of relatively superficial behavioral difficulties, just as they were critical of their total situation. At that time Carl's grades did not reflect any decline in school behavior or performance. Indeed his playground behavior seemed decidedly improved.

The social worker's notes commented that the mother had been unable to follow-up on the previous suggestions made in the absence of therapeutic contact for herself. Consequently she gave the mother information about other sources of help available and recommended that the family seek additional treatment. (Despite her earlier efforts to involve the father, the clinician obviously ended up dealing with the mother.)

Case 3: Grade Change, − 0.87; Playground Rating Change, + 1.55

Dorothy, an 11 year old girl, was the only child of a Hi SEL family; the recent (2 year) marriage was the mother's second. Referral Category: Social Withdrawal moderate severity. Ammons IQ = 140.

SCHOOL REFERRAL DATA

"Selects only one friend; aloof, withdrawn, sensitive, very quiet, appears docile. Mother was most responsive to suggestion of referral; is eager for help and feels very unable to understand her daughter."

* Quotes are from the progress notes in the clinic records.

TREATMENT FORMAT

Female counselor, expert. Ten family discussions covering a wide range of content and feeling revealed great conflict in the family, especially between daughter and stepfather. There was a very close, ambivalent relationship between mother and daughter. Testing suggested fairly severe emotional and social difficulties in this young girl, so at termination of the (already extended) social work sessions, referral for additional help was made.

FOLLOW-UP

The family came in readily for three follow-up interviews and continued to seek a variety of kinds of psychological treatment over the years. The parents participated for a long period in a marital counseling group conducted by a psychologist in private practice; the daughter entered individual psychotherapy with a psychiatrist but soon refused to continue. When she entered junior high school her school and social life were continuing to deteriorate. At one point the parents called the clinic to ask help in hospitalizing her: Her behavior at home had been openly hostile and her mother felt the daughter had threatened her with a knife. A psychiatric evaluation resulted in a recommendation that Dorothy be placed in a residential treatment center, but the mother then repudiated this move. The crisis subsided and Dorothy was placed in a private day school where she gradually established an adequate school and social adjustment. This occurred after the second follow-up interview. By this time the marital conflict was the major focus of family attention and by the time of the third follow-up (2 years after completion of clinic treatment) the mother was seeking individual therapy for herself.

According to the case record, the Parent Counseling hours were focused on the total family situation and relationships, not on specific behavior of the girl. Dorothy's improvement on the playground ($+1.55$) is interesting in view of the fact that it was ultimately through her peer relationships that she apparently attained some psychological equilibrium.

Parent Counseling Summary

The presence of a new stepfather in the home led to refusal of treatment for one child whose grades improved without clinical intervention. An intact black family's child showed gradual and consistent grade improvement after parents were assured of his basic learning capacity, despite fluctuations in their tolerance for his occasional difficulties. The record indicates that the focus of parental concern shifted from its initial emphasis on the child's potential disability to more general family problems. In the unimproved case, long continuing animosity between a stepfather and daughter was basically untouched by more than 3 years of various types of psychological and psychiatric treatment: improvement came only when the girl was old enough to separate herself psychologically from the parents and establish meaningful peer relationships.

Referral for additional treatment occurred in cases in which the grades criterion reflected improvement as well as in unimproved cases, though help was most often sought for others in the family, at the later times.

CHILD THERAPY

Case 1: Grade Change, +0.75

Greg was 9 years old, from a Hi SEL, intact family; he had one sister, aged 7. He had a history of asthma and hypoglycemia which was controlled largely by diet. He had nightmares and was given tranquilizing pills at bedtime (prescribed by the pediatrician). Referral Category: Attention Control, moderate severity.

SCHOOL REFERRAL DATA

School personnel reported reading difficulties, poor work habits, distractibility, and nonacceptance by peers. The youngster was not a source of major concern to the school, but the principal noted that the mother was insistent that the child be referred to the clinic for treatment.

FAMILY

Both parents were college graduates; the father, 35, was a professional man who described himself as a "man of few words." His wife described him as a "volcano that periodically erupts." He stated that he was not permitted by his wife to discipline his son; she claimed he was unduly rough and harsh in his discipline. The mother was depicted in the record as anxious, overtalkative, and overprotective. She "hates housework" and the house was often "quite a shambles." She was very active in church work, scouting activities, and the PTA.

TREATMENT FORMAT

Female therapist, social worker, expert. Treatment was discontinued by the mother after the fourth (of 20 allotted) sessions, reputedly because the therapist had discussed sex with the child. Therapy notes quoted the mother as fuming that she had brought her son to the clinic "for his reading problem and not for birth information." There had been one family session and each parent had been seen once. The therapist noted that the mother had appeared controlling and competitive from the outset. The child, in contrast, had related warmly to her and had been free in his communication. His self-image was that of being "bruised and cut up"; he identified strongly with his mother; he had extreme curiosity along with his inability to read, to find out; his younger sister was "the enemy." Other treatment notes indicate that the youngster's main defenses were displacement, reaction formation, and projection.

FOLLOW-UP

When the family was offered a follow-up appointment by the original clinician, the mother was very pleasant but refused the appointment because the boy had recently tripped and fallen, breaking both legs and one arm. He was in casts and would be in bed for several months. He was getting individual tutoring as a consequence of being bedridden. The mother reported being very pleased with this teaching arrangement. She had transferred him from the referring public school to a private school since leaving the clinic, but was not sure where she would reenter him after his recovery.

Case 2: Grade Change, +0.69

Julian was an 8 year old boy, an only child living with his mother and stepfather. Lo SEL; black; they rented a two-bedroom home. Referral Category: Hyperactivity, low degree of severity.

SCHOOL REFERRAL DATA

"Does not tolerate long periods in classroom; does very little work; has difficulty getting along with other children."

FAMILY

Stepfather, 40, was a waiter; the mother, 42, a dry-cleaning checker. They had been married for only a few months. Both had moved to the Los Angeles area in the last couple of years. The mother saw Julian's problem as due to lack of discipline resulting from her failure to set limits during the years she lived alone with her son. Both parents expressed themselves as agreeable, and even enthusiastic, about coming to the clinic.

TREATMENT FORMAT

Male therapist, psychologist, expert. Twelve individual therapy sessions were held with the boy, following one family intake; there were three cancellations even though transportation was supplied by university car. There was no follow-up interview.

The therapist's treatment notes focus on the child's anger and his general problem relative to the expression of aggression. There was modeling and discussion of limit setting, along with fostering of appropriate channels for expression of feeling. Notes report the child's pride when realizing he could express himself while at the same time taking responsibility for his actions. The therapist's impressions were that the youngster was achieving more constructive modes for expression of his anger; for example, he was taking pride in not hurting himself when angry and he was starting to incorporate the therapist's attitude toward expression of feeling insofar as freedom and limits were concerned.

In his summary the psychologist noted that Julian remained quite an angry child who would need repeated consistent experience in implementing what he had learned. He expressed the hope that the mother would now be better able to provide this structure for her son. (This suggests that the stepfather was not playing a very active role with his new son.)

FOLLOW-UP

Very shortly after termination, the school doctor and nurse contacted the clinic to express concern about the boy's failure to pay attention in class, his short attention span, poor performance, and occasional falling asleep in the classroom. They sought suggestions for handling these problems. The therapist, when contacted, felt the difficulties were closely related to the problems in expression of aggression and made some general suggestions relative to modes of supervision which might help the youngster and the school. The family could not be located for a follow-up interview at 6 months past treatment's end.

Case 3: Grade Change, − 0.87

Louise was 11 years old, with two younger siblings in an intact Hi SEL family; they owned their three-bedroom home. Referral Category: Attention Control, low severity.

SCHOOL REFERRAL DATA

School personnel noted some rebelliousness and insolence; her performance in all areas was going down; she "seemed different." Parents were delighted to receive psychological help, as they felt they could not cope with their daughter.

FAMILY

Father, 34, was an insurance broker with junior college background; mother, 33, was a housewife with one semester of college. Complaints about the daughter included "sexual precocity" (when the parents had been away on vacation she had had dates), some instances of pilfering, and *much* glibness and lying; they never knew when to believe her. There was conflict between the daughter and each of the other family members.

TREATMENT FORMAT

Female therapist, psychologist, expert. Intake plus 12 therapy sessions (seven with daughter, three with parents and daughter, two with parents; one follow-up; no missed or cancelled appointments).

Treatment notes focused on the therapist's interpretations of behavior and relationships (oedipal material, indications of transference, etc.). These were mostly not verbalized to the family, apparently, though some interpretations were occasionally suggested in individual sessions with the girl (who appears from the notes to have remained quiet and seemingly unresponsive). Areas of conflict between all family members were gradually made explicit in discussions during the therapy series. The therapist felt that the parents were too permissive and made suggestions as to ways in which they could require more cooperation and responsibility on their daughter's part. She also worked to have the parents become aware of the interpersonal manipulations of the daughter.

Treatment notes indicated that the parents were more relaxed at the end of therapy and there were signs of improving cooperation on the girl's part.

FOLLOW-UP

Parents had been feeling much better about their daughter and much more in control, but a report card brought home the week of the third follow-up appointment revealed a marked decline in Louise's grades. The parents were greatly upset by this but the therapist felt that even so, they were less swayed by their daughter's cunning and were taking more active responsibility for her behavior.

Two years later the clinic received a request for information on our contacts with this family from the daughter's junior high school.

Case 4: Grade Change, − 1.25

Dave, 11, had one sister aged 17. There were two older brothers who were out of the home. The mother had been divorced for 7 years. Hi SEL; they owned their three-bedroom home but currently the family was in extreme financial distress and the mortgage on the home was being foreclosed. Referral Category: Hyperactivity, low degree of severity.

SCHOOL REFERRAL DATA

"Trouble at school, mostly talking when he shouldn't; talks back; doesn't do as he is told; doesn't respect authority; doesn't get along with peers."

FAMILY

Mother, 40, high school graduate, had no vocation. She considered her middle name "unlucky," was always getting into accidents and troubles, was an easy victim for "con artists." The daughter was quiet, mature, and responsible. Dave spent 1 year in a military school and had stayed for long periods with various relatives. He declared his love for his mother but had many complaints about her.

TREATMENT FORMAT

Male therapist, psychologist, expert. Intake plus 12 therapy sessions; one missed appointment. The therapist's notes indicate brief contacts with mother at the start of some hours, but the major focus was explicitly kept on the boy. Content of hours centered around the boy's sadness and loneliness, also around his frustration with his mother, toward whom he felt both anger and protectiveness. Over the sessions his complaints about her grew angrier. He seemed to enjoy his sessions, especially the checker games and candy involved in them. Though his school misbehavior continued, he expressed attachment for the therapist and did not want the sessions to end. Treatment involved considerable work on insight into his ambivalent feelings and needs in many areas. The mother continued to be caught up in catastrophies and the school felt that both the boy's behavior and his life situation were deteriorating. The principal called the therapist to discuss the possibility of having the boy placed outside the home. The mother vacillated on this and the therapist spent some time trying to clarify her feelings; he also explored with her some financial moves and resources open to her. At termination several referrals and alternatives were discussed.

There was no follow-up with this family, but a year later we received an inquiry about the boy from a local institution at which the mother was seeking placement for her son.

Case 5: Grade Change, −1.25; Playground Rating Change, +2.35

Tom was a 10 year old boy with a twice-divorced mother and an older brother aged 12. Mid SEL: rented apartment. Referral Category: Attention Control, moderate severity.

SCHOOL REFERRAL DATA

"Great need for attention which he seeks in undesirable ways; appears to lack self-control; requires an unusual amount of motivation to complete assignments."

FAMILY

Mother, 30, a bookkeeper with a high school education, declared herself eager for help with her son with whom she had much conflict. The stepfather from whom she had been separated for 3 years had explicitly preferred the older boy.

TREATMENT FORMAT

Male therapist, psychologist, expert. Intake plus 12 therapy sessions; 17 missed and cancelled appointments; one follow-up. The treatment series was maintained despite the irregular attendance because there seemed to be indications of improvement in the boy's grades and behavior during the treatment and his mother reported that he was always worse when they missed an appointment at the clinic. The youngster himself spoke of feeling and behaving better and evidenced real affection for the therapist and a desire to continue seeing him. Treatment dealt with his angry feelings toward his mother, his increasing needs for autonomy on the one hand, and his defeatist self-concept and feelings of depression on the other.

FOLLOW-UP

At the 6 month follow-up which occurred early in September, the therapist recorded the mother's reports of continued improvement at school (though the boy had not been in school over the summer). She felt he had improved considerably and was more positive in his approach, for example, "He no longer feels that he's stupid but rather that he can cope." During the hour a charge-countercharge conflict built up between mother and son, suggesting to the therapist that their differences were occurring on a more overt level. Statements at the end of the session were described as quite positive in all respects. They were scheduled for a second follow-up but failed to appear. Shortly before that, the family had moved and the boy had been suspended from a new school. The new principal called the clinic stating that the suspension was an effort to force the mother to return the boy for help; school personnel believed he needed to be hospitalized. The mother kept one appointment at this time but was mainly preoccupied with the loss of her recent boyfriend. She was referred for help for herself and the boy to a mental health facility in their new community.

Child Therapy Summary

Parents of two of the three children whose grades improved most in this group had discontinued psychotherapeutic treatment of the child in the early stages. Parental jealousy of the potential influence of the therapist is at least one possible reason for the parents' rejection of this treatment modality. Among the cases whose grades dropped, one had minimal signs of clinical improvement in the record; the other two cases came from chaotic situations that would certainly have had poor prognosis for benefit from any treatment. It may be significant, however, that both these cases were boys who had had almost no paternal figure in their lives and both were seen by a male therapist. In view of the critical role fathers seem to represent for boys at this age level, the speculation arises as to whether such limited exposure to an involved male therapist may not increase the boy's awareness of emotional needs for a father and, in turn, increase his desperation, acting out, and disturbance, at least temporarily.

A reading of the Child Therapy and Parent Counseling records suggested that these two treatments often differed primarily in number of sessions. Otherwise many interviews seemed quite similar in style and content. Some Parent Counseling sessions seemed more focused on specific problems, whereas many therapy hours were more oriented to emotional exploration involving broader parental and familial areas. This latter approach might well open up more diffuse and complex problems; these would seem less amenable to short-term intervention. Referrals for additional treatment were offered (and often sought by parents) at the conclusion of both these interventions.

CHAPTER 10

The Information Feedback Intervention

The Information Feedback procedures had a number of specific goals which are summarized below. The techniques, the examples, and process measures that follow show how we attempted to implement these goals.*

1. Attention was directed toward the interpersonal plane: toward interpersonal perceptions, communication processes, and interactions *between* people. This perspective was expected to be less threatening to self-esteem than focus on actions which ascribe guilt or responsibility to individuals. It should therefore arouse less avoidant or other defensive reactions.

2. Objective scrutiny of behavior was promoted. Attention was directed toward external manifestations of the way communications or interactions look or sound, rather than to any intent implied by or assumed for the behavior. In this way, sources of interpersonal differences in perception could be identified by participants and a common frame of reference established.

3. Efforts were made to encourage explicit discrimination of behaviors, without necessarily minimizing affective reactions. It was assumed that behavior which could be related to identified stimulus sources was likely to seem relatively understandable and potentially controllable.

4. A process of scanning the interpersonal environment was facilitated. This would include as complete a range of information about people's behavior as possible, in order to increase the probability that different observers would respond to the greatest possible overlap of behavioral information. The survey was also intended to provide new evidence that is confirming and gratifying about interactions, as well as unearthing differences that require resolution.

5. Particularly through playback of the videotapes, Information Feedback attempted to increase the salience of nonverbal communications. These typically receive scant attention in the context of the socially emphasized verbal aspects of communication.

---

* Portions of these materials are also reported in Kaswan, Love, and Rodnick (1971).
© 1971 by Academic Press, Inc. and reprinted by permission.

6. Finally, a major goal was to place primary reliance on the family's own problem-solving abilities. To whatever extent they were able to improve their own situation, parents were presumed to be simultaneously developing greater feelings of competence and solidarity within the family unit. To the extent that the emotional investment of trust and dependency was maintained within the family group, instead of being shifted to a clinician, there should be significant emotional gain for initiative and coherence within the family.

There is no claim that these goals could be applied realistically to extremely severe impairment of behavior. They seemed applicable, however, to the broad range of children's problems customarily encountered in the family and school difficulties described in this report.

DESCRIPTION OF THE INTERVENTION

Clinic personnel involved in the Information Feedback intervention included two consultants for each family, one responsible for contacts with the adults, one for the often simultaneous but separate contacts with the child. Two or three research assistants (depending on family size) administered measures, handled TV playbacks, supplied child care, etc. The involvement of several people was planned to avoid any implied encouragement of a traditionally confidential, one-to-one therapeutic relationship. Efforts were made to establish a friendly but business-like atmosphere. To this end a number of standard "spiels" were used by all personnel in introducing and discussing the goals and techniques of the project. These were not quoted verbatim but each consultant stayed as close to the prescribed format as he could without sounding stiff or artificial.

In order to acquaint families with our use of videotapes, and also to further standardize the orientation they received to our goals, we used a prepared videotape in which the feedback approach was described. Consultants played this tape for each family in the first interview, immediately after the family interactions had been videorecorded and the initial adjective ratings of family members had been completed. The transcript of the tape is as follows:

I am Dr. Barthol.* I would like to describe some of the things we do here. You will get more details later, but we like everyone to get a general picture of our approach right at the outset.

* We are grateful to Dr. Richard Barthol, Professor of Psychology, UCLA, for this important contribution. He was not otherwise involved in any of the procedures.

Most of the families come here because one or more of their children have problems at school and often at home. In working on such problems we have developed an approach which many people find they can use to make whatever changes they want. For the most part, this approach helps you to take a fresh look at how you and the child talk and behave with each other. For example, how often are you sure that your child (or someone else in your family) really knows what you mean when you talk with them? How often are you sure that *you* understand what they are trying to say to you? Questions like these are especially important when a child is not doing as well as he should. Since he spends most of his time at home or at school, his family and the teacher are usually the most important people in his life and are the ones best able to help him. For this reason, the first job is to find out exactly how you and the child actually see and relate to each other. This is the object of much of our work here and we have special ways to help to sharpen your eyes and ears as you look at and talk with each other. Some of the things you did here today were part of this work.

So that we can get a better picture of how your family acts, we will also visit you at home. Along the way, different members of the family may get some tests which give information about people's abilities and ways of approaching problems. Since many of the child's difficulties may show up in school, we have visited there to talk with the teacher and have seen your child in his classroom and on the playground.

During the ten or twelve weeks we will be working together you will be looking at all this information about your child, your family, and your child's school situation. Once you have this information, it is likely that you will see ways of handling these problems on your own, just as you handle other important problems in your daily life.

In general, then, our approach is to help you get more facts, leaving it up to you how to use them to best help your child.

Families had a number of reactions to the videotaped description. Negative reactions focused on parental expectations and needs to get *help*, to receive guidance as to what they should do. Some parents seemed both frightened and resentful that quick professional answers would not be forthcoming, or that the child was not going to receive "treatment" that should change him. Positive reactions reflected approval and apparent relief that intimate emotional explorations were not going to be required, that the focus might stay on their presenting problem, the child, without shifting to parental, personal, or marital conflicts. As indicated previously, it was generally felt that fathers responded more positively to this initial description of the approach than mothers did.

In all cases, the TV presentation was very effective in getting everyone's attention. It stimulated discussion about interactions in the family, usually centering on the child's problems. After this, the parents and target child participated in the Family Communication Task which directed attention specifically to the effectiveness of communication within the family. Parents were then given copies of the Behavior Inventory to take home and an appointment was made for two project members to visit the home during the following week at a time when everyone would be present.

The home visit was planned to permit observation of family interactions in their natural setting. Our difficulties in getting reliable data in this setting are described in the next chapter.

The next three or four meetings with the family were held in the clinic and constituted the core of the feedback intervention. At each appointment, material that the consultants had gathered previously was presented to the family. The first feedback was of the Family Adjective Ratings. Composite graphs showing the ratings of all three members, each represented by a differently colored profile, were prepared for all concepts selected for feedback. For example, one composite sheet contained the father's profiled ratings of "myself," the mother's of "my spouse," and the child's of "my father"; the three perceptions of the father were then compared and discussed. Comparisons similarly were translated into visual terms for mother's rating of "how my child will rate me" with the child's actual rating of "my mother." Concerns about how people appeared to each other were consistently indicated in their active interest in studying the juxtaposed profiles. The process usually started out with a good deal of laughter and joking but settled quickly into careful scrutiny, often with considerable anxiety. Surprise was almost always expressed at some point or other in the family comparison, often with intensity. One upper-middle-class mother appeared genuinely startled to discover that her high ratings on "bored" for herself were matched by high ratings on "angry" in her husband's and child's perceptions of her, and that her expectation of high ratings on "friendly" were not realized.

The method and content of all feedback sessions were designed to keep each person actively evaluating what he heard and saw. Each person's perception was specified (through a rating) and made public (ratings had been graphed and sets of graphs were compared openly) so that differences and verifications could constantly occur.

At the second clinic appointment, after they had considered and discussed graphs of their Family Adjective Ratings, each parent and the target child separately viewed selected brief scenes from the family videotape. Each made individual adjective ratings of a set of concepts such as "Helen in relation to the family," for each scene. Standard instructions were given to look at the videotape "as if you were looking at strangers; look at it the way someone would who did not know the people involved." They were also reminded that they would later have an opportunity to compare their ratings with those of project raters who knew nothing about their family. These instructions hopefully focused people's attention on objective behavior (e.g., how it *looks* or *sounds* to others) rather than on anyone's interpretation of what someone "meant" or "intended." At the third session, prepared graphs which reflected agreements and disagreements in the different sets of ratings of the scenes were shown to the family.

The selection of scenes for rating were made by the consultants and included excerpts from total family interactions as well as the dyad periods. There were always at least two scenes from the problem definition. The scenes were from 30 to 90 seconds long, the objective being to capture a brief episode with a clearly defined beginning and end. They were selected from about the middle of each type of interaction, provided the people involved were understandable and in camera range.

After ratings of all excerpts had been discussed, the family was shown the total videotape. The tape could be stopped for discussion at any point, and much feeling was often expressed during the viewing. "I never knew I looked so mad" was a typical response. It was made several times by the same mother who had rated herself as bored on the FARS but had been seen as "angry" and unfriendly by her family.

The excerpted scenes had been rated first in order to direct attention to specific behaviors, before the affective context of being observed had been reinstituted. This was again an attempt to maximize the objectivity with which the excerpts could be viewed.

Children were present at feedback sessions at the parent's option. In most cases they were not only there, but participated with apparent interest and comprehension in these quite complex activities, though age and IQ factors had to be kept constantly in mind. When material was carefully chosen and geared at appropriate levels, however, children seemed intrigued, not only with videotapes, but with interpersonal phenomena in general. The consultants selected material for feedback to sample the range of family behavior, as there was obviously too much material for total coverage. Choices were supposed to be made on the basis of the representativeness of the family behaviors, rather than with the goal of highlighting behaviors that seemed to the consultant to need changing.

Similar visual presentation was made of data from the Family Communication Task and the Behavior Inventories. In all sessions, the consultant's role was to direct the attention and discussion of family members to their own recorded and rated behavior. Apart from emphasizing this consistent focus, he attempted to avoid interpretation, suggestion, reflection, or other therapeutic techniques. Needless to say, there was variation in consultant ability to restructure their usual clinical role in this way, but this was an explicit orientation accepted by each consultant. (A general problem for these clinicians was a tendency to appear somewhat stiff and distant, in their attempts to be impersonal and atherapeutic.)

A feedback session with comparable material was provided for school personnel at the clinic. Teachers were shown graphs of their ratings of the target child in comparison with their view of the average child, of their perception of the "average" child at that grade level with other (anonymous) teachers' ratings of children at this level, etc. They viewed profiles reflecting the differences between their expectations as to how the child would rate them with the child's actual ratings. Within the limits determined by individual parental approval, selected material from family data was made available. Similarities and differences in Teacher and Parent Behavior Inventory items were profiled for teachers, just as they had been for parents, to point up significant differences in perceptions and expectations of the child at home and school.

The final meeting was held at the school and involved the parents, the teacher, the principal, the counselor, and a project staff member in his role as consultant. Since the school staff had originally referred the child to the clinic because of problems which they identified, this final session provided an appropriate opportunity for school personnel to review the original problem with the parents in light of information obtained in the project. They could make joint plans for working together in handling the child's difficulty. The consultant served as a source of information but refrained from offering specific suggestions.

Examples follow which illustrate the feedback of adjective ratings and behavior inventories with individual cases.

Figure 12 is an example of a profile composite used in one feedback session. It illustrates how the mother, father, child, and two neutral observers (Raters 1 and 2) had rated the mother's behavior in one of six scenes selected by the consultant as representative of the family's videotaped interactions.

The child in this case was an 11 year old boy adopted in infancy, the only child of parents in their late 40s. He was referred because both the school and parents were concerned about his general immaturity and what they considered to be his extremely effeminate behavior and interests. The parents were also disturbed by his passive but effective resistance to their discipline and his failure to take on responsibilities appropriate to his age.

The scene that was rated was taken from an early part of the free family interaction. At the beginning of this scene, the mother was busy at the refreshment table arranging juice and cookies (in contrast to the patterns for most families in which each member helped himself). The child was winding the spinning top nearby; the father was sitting in a chair. The scene lasted 70 seconds and consisted of the following interaction:

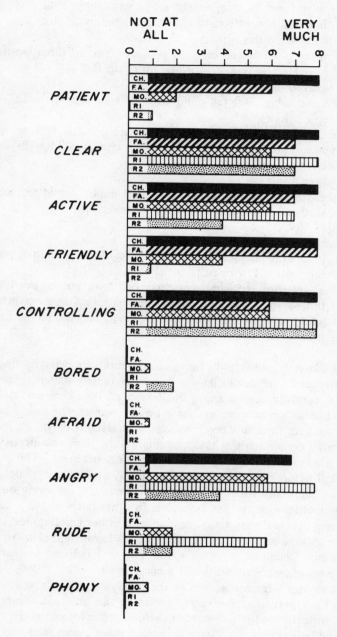

Figure 12. Composite profile of TV ratings as used in feedback sessions.

Mo: Bill, you are not listening [child plays with top]. You don't have much time and I want you to eat (mother points to chair).

Ch: I just want to do this top.

Mo: Want me to put this one here, so you can (two or three words not clear). . . Here is you . . . Now, hurry up Bill . . .

Ch: I just want to finish this.

Fa: Not on the table, Bill [as child tries to spin top on table—child spins top on floor].

Mo: Come on, I want you to get started, you are going to be hungry and then you are going to cry [hands juice to child—child spills some].

Mo: See, there you are—see?

Fa: How about wiping it now.

Mo: See, see, what you carry on? [Mother gets napkin, child reaches out for it. Mother brushes it over his hand, bends down.]

Fa: Let him wipe it.

Ch: Let me wipe it.

Fa: Put it [cup with juice] down, put the thing down. [Child wipes up, apparently only a few drips.]

Mo: [as child gets up] See what you carry on? Now go on, put it away [child throws juice container into trash barrel]. Come on now, sit down [child sits down]. Here you are now, be careful [as mother hands him juice, napkin, cookies].

Figure 12 shows that the child's ratings of the mother's behavior fluctuate between extremes on the scale: he saw her as extremely patient, clear, active, friendly, controlling, and angry but not at all bored, afraid, rude, or phony. This fluctuation between extremes (which was usually found in children much younger than this boy) was quite characteristic of his ratings. The father rated the mother's behavior as high on the positive adjectives but his ratings also reflected her general controlling behavior. The mother marked herself as having little patience, being only moderately friendly, and seeming quite angry and rude. This particular scene is a relatively mild example of the mother's controlling behavior. In other parts of the videotape her dominating is revealed to be more emphatic in her cajoling and threats (e.g., "I'll never do another thing for you"; "Let's leave right now"). (During the Problem Definition discussion, this boy was reduced to tears and screams by both parents' criticisms and accusations.)

When the ratings were first shown to the family, all three began actively to compare their perceptions of each person in the different scenes. The mother said little during these discussions although she looked at the ratings carefully. The father, perhaps after seeing the mother's own relatively negative evaluation of her behavior, began to be very critical of her. After about

5 minutes of his criticism, during which the mother seemed very uncomfortable, she said, "Of course, I can see that's not the way to do things. I can see for myself after all." The father softened his remarks and the mother later asked to take the ratings home (as did many other families).

In this, as in many other cases, it was our impression that the ratings were not only a way of recording perceptions but also provided a relatively impersonal device through which the family could identify and communicate their perceptions of each other, thus creating a basis for improved understanding. Viewing the ratings of the two neutral observers also helped to decrease the threat inherent in negative evaluations by other members of the family. As an indication of such reduced defensiveness, this pair of parents began to perceive their own behavior as evoking the very behaviors in their son to which they most objected. In particular, they recognized the effect of their overcontrolling behavior and began to help him accept more individual responsibility. The school personnel also responded with interest to increased information about this boy. When he was to leave elementary school for junior high, the principal took the initiative and expended much time in arranging for Bill to be allowed to go to a different school than his residence would dictate, in order that he not be separated from two boys with whom he had recently established friendly relationships.

The Parent and Teacher Behavior Inventories provided another device for encouraging the differentiation of actual behavior from generalized expectations. They thus served to objectify judgments and direct attention to behavioral characteristics and consequences.

The format and use of the Parent Behavior Inventory is illustrated by an example (Figure 13). Items on this page deal with the parents' activities with the child. The mother's ratings are indicated with an "M," the father's with an "F."

The 9 year old boy in this family was referred because he frequently disturbed the classroom, teased other children into attacking him, and showed visible self-mutilating behavior. Although he was of above-average intelligence, he was a nonreader and was retarded by at least a year in other academic subjects. When given individual attention, however, he performed well and seemed anxious to please. The parents were aware of problems at school, but reported no serious difficulties at home, except for the self-mutilation. The parents said very little when they looked at the various rating profiles and videotapes. After examining the Behavior Inventory (which they took home to consider further) the mother commented, ". . . It doesn't look like we have much to do with him . . . I guess we don't show him much feeling. I wonder if he needs some . . ." No comments from the consultant were called for or expected. Like many others who participated in the project, these parents were unsophisticated people with less than high

13. How often do you do the following with your child:

	At most several times a year	About once a month	About once a week	Almost every day	Several times a day
(a) Go camping, picnicking or on trips		F M			
(b) Go to movies, sports, etc.	F M				
(c) Play ball or other sports			F M		
(d) Wrestle, roughhouse		F M			
(e) Play quiet games (like checkers, cards)					

(f) Watch television together

(g) Read to him

(h) Help with homework

(i) Teach him new things

	At most several times a year	About once a month	About once a week	Almost every day	Several times a day
(f) Watch television together	F				
(g) Read to him	F M				
(h) Help with homework	F	M			
(i) Teach him new things	F	M			

19. How much time do you and your child usually spend together when you are at home evenings?

Rarely have any time	A few minutes	About an hour	Two or more hours
		F M	

20. How many nights during the week are you usually at home before your child goes to sleep?

0-1	2-3	4-5	6-7
F		M	

21. How much time do you spend in some activity with your children on weekends?

Rarely have any time	An occasional hour	At least one hour each weekend	Several hours a weekend

Fig. 13. Sample page of Parent Behavior Inventory prepared for feedback to parents.

Child Study Program
Psychology – UCLA

68. How often do you do the following when your child quarrels or fights with other children:

	At most several times a year	About once a month	About once a week	Almost every day	Several times a day
(c) Step in if fighting gets rough			F	M	
(d) Punish the child for fighting			F	M	
(e) Talk with the other parents about the children's fighting	F		M		

69. To what extent does your child quarrel or fight with his brothers and sisters?

At most several times a year	About once a month	About once a week	Almost every day	Several times a day
		F	M	

70. How often do you do the following when your child quarrels with his brothers and sisters:

	At most several times a year	About once a month	About once a week	Almost every day	Several times a day
(a) Leave them alone			F	M	

212

	At most several times a year	About once a month	About once a week	Almost every day	Several times a day
(b) Step in before a real fight starts			*E*	*M*	
(c) Step in only if fighting gets violent		*F*	*M*		
(d) Punish the child for fighting					

7. How often does your child decide:

	At most several times a year	About once a month	About once a week	Almost every day	Several times a day
(a) What he should wear				*M* *F*	
(b) When he should do his homework			*F*	*M*	
(c) Who he can have as friends					*M* *F*

Figure 13. (Continued)

school education and no previous contact with mental health agencies. Their child's school grades improved more than in any other case: this is child # 1, Information Feedback, presented in Chapter 9.

A final example involves a child's dramatic change in behavior that appeared to be in direct relationship to the TV viewing. This 10 year old girl had manifested highly atypical behavior at several points in the family room interaction. This consisted of shrill giggles, frenetic (autistic-like) hand movements, momentary gibber-type verbalization, and a peculiar repeated jabbing at the blackboard with chalk. Whenever this occurred her parents interrupted their usual preoccupation with the two younger male siblings to admonish her severely, threaten her with spankings, exclusion, and the like. In viewing the total videotape both parents (but the father especially) quickly noted the attention-getting quality of the girl's behavior. (In her preschool years she had been under psychiatric treatment and on medication for several years. She had been able to attend public school but had always been a social isolate, a scapegoat for children's taunts because of the mannerisms which appeared when she was upset.) When the child herself initially viewed an excerpt containing this behavior, she was in a separate room with the consultant, rating the excerpts. Her attention seemed literally riveted to the peculiar behavior. She appeared surprised and embarrassed and after a moment went into a long rationalized explanation of why she had done something so "silly." When she later saw this behavior while viewing the entire tape in the presence of the total family, she immediately exploded into a frenzied repetition of the behavior. Her outburst became so extreme that the viewing had to be interrupted temporarily. Later she asked the consultant if she might see that section of the tape again. At each clinic visit thereafter she repeated this request; it was granted whenever time permitted. Reports from the school indicated that this behavior (which had previously been characteristic at school as well) disappeared immediately and did not recur. Apparently her behavior at home also improved gradually because she was allowed new privileges and activities (e.g., an overnight camping trip with a scout troop, the kind of thing her mother had not previously permitted on the grounds that the girl couldn't take care of herself, she was too silly, too babyish, etc.). At about this time her father brought home, as a surprise, a new bedroom set for her room. He comforted her when she broke into tears, and effectively stopped the mother from admonishing her for again being babyish.

It was the impression of the clinic team working with this family that this was a clear-cut example of a child's indentification of objectively undesirable behavior in herself, and her immediate substitution of other, more adaptive behaviors. Despite the fact that the behavior in question was so bizarre as to be almost pathognomic (it was immediately identified as autistic-like by all clinicians viewing the videotape), she was still able to suppress it effectively in the school setting within a period of about 2 weeks. It tapered off at home as well, though more slowly and less dramatically. It should be noted that in granting the child's request to review that part of the videotape, the consultant did not discuss the recorded behavior with her, or her reasons for wanting to look at it. This family was followed over a 2 year period, with continuing progress being shown by all family members.

DATA REFLECTING THE CHANGE PROCESS

Though our treatment groups were very small we have analyzed process data wherever possible. These are presented only as tentative indications of the way in which we see the change process occurring in this type of intervention.

Family Ratings of TV Excerpts

The 30 families receiving the Information Feedback intervention and the 29 control families rated brief scenes from their family videotapes. As described, family members were instructed to be as objective as possible and to rate the specific behaviors recorded. These ratings were compared with the general ratings the family members had made of themselves and eachother (FARS, Chapter 3). In the TV ratings, the Information Feedback subgroup of the R families rated much more like the NR families than they had in general family ratings (FARS). Analysis of their TV ratings (Appendix B, Tables 25, 26, 27, and 28) show few significant R/NR group differences. This change seems reasonable in terms of the situational constraints that were common to the setting for both parents, but it may also reflect the instructions given the Information Feedback families to be objective in their ratings.

In rating the videotapes, R mothers' ratings seem to reflect a more positive appraisal of husband and child, and a less positive view of the self than their FARS results had indicated. Similarly, the videotaped behavior of both sets of mothers was rated by all the family as equal on negativity, and lower in Positive Impact than either fathers or children, in contrast to the high social effectiveness attributed to the mothers by R fathers and children on the FARS (Chapter 3).

The two groups of fathers continued to be rated differently by their families, in the TV excerpts as in the FARS, with favorableness always attributed to the NR. In their own ratings, however, R fathers apparently rated themselves and their families very like the ratings made by NR fathers.

Though this is only descriptive material, it is at least consistent with the repeated comments by observers that Information Feedback fathers tended to be pleasantly surprised on viewing the videotapes, in contrast to their wives who seemed to react with discomfort.

These ratings indicate that the two sets of fathers and mothers viewed and were viewed in the TV excerpts in the same general terms that the project raters used in their detailed sequential ratings (Chapter 4). It was hoped that the instructions facilitated objective self- and other appraisals within the family, and provided a reasonably nonjudgmental atmosphere in which changes might be considered.

Pre-Post Changes in Information Feedback Families

CHANGES IN VIDEOTAPED FAMILY INTERACTION

Changes from original to follow-up clinic visits were examined on all comparisons which had yielded significant differences between referred and nonreferred groups in the analysis of the initial videotaped interaction (see Chapter 4). These included:

1. Expressive extremes of father behavior: referred fathers were rated as appearing extremely positive or negative (or both) in comparison to nonreferred fathers.
2. Expressive extremes of child behavior: referred children were rated as appearing extremely positive or negative (or both) in comparison to nonreferred children.
3. Directing behavior of fathers: referred fathers were seen as more directive than nonreferred fathers.
4. Talkativeness of fathers: referred fathers talked more than nonreferred fathers.

Follow-up tapes were available for only 10 of the 20 referred families in this sample whose initial interaction had been studied in detail (see Chapter 4). In view of the small number of cases, the results reported below must be considered only illustrative of the processes believed to occur in response to the Information Feedback experiences.

Pre-post treatment comparisons were made between families receiving Information Feedback ($N = 4$) and families receiving Parent Counseling or Child Therapy ($N = 6$). Evaluative range* (our measure of affective extremes; see Chapter 4) appears to have decreased somewhat more for fa-

---

* Evaluative variability was measured for equivalent time periods (free interaction and problem definition of original and follow-up tapes).

thers and children after Information Feedback than for fathers and children who had received either of the other treatments (see Figure 14; F Group $\times$ Time $= 4.83; df = 1,5; p < .10$, Appendix B, Table 29).

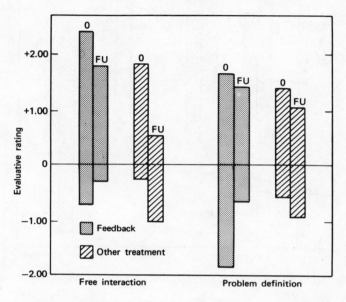

Figure 14. Father's evaluative range at intake (O) and at follow-up (FU).

Separate analyses of positive and negative extremes of evaluative range revealed different change patterns for different treatment groups. There was no significant Group $\times$ Time interaction for positive extremes, because all fathers tended to decrease in these. However, for negative extremes, the Group $\times$ Times interaction yields an $F = 8.67; df = 1,5; p < .05$. As Figure 14 shows, fathers receiving Information Feedback decreased in negative extremes. Fathers in other treatment groups, on the other hand, became *more* extreme in their negative behavior. It should be noted that the follow-up situation was different for the feedback families because they had seen their initial interaction videotapes, while the other families had not.

Children in the Information Feedback group decreased in both positive and negative extremes. Children in other groups, however, *increased* in positive extremes and showed an uneven change pattern for negative extremes (see Figure 15). [For evaluative range (both extremes), the Group $\times$ Time interaction was $F = 9.23; df = 1/8; p < .05$, Appendix B, Table 30. For the positive extreme, the Group $\times$ Time interaction was $F = 5.84; df = 1/8; p < .05.$] Positive evaluative extremes in children had been in-

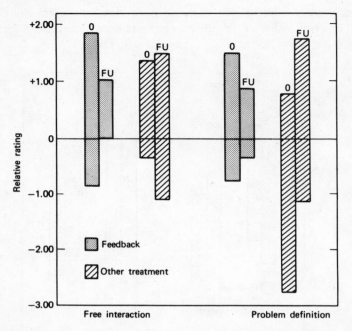

Figure 15.   Children's evaluative range at intake (O) and at follow-up (FU).

terpreted in our original tape analysis (Chapter 4) as reflecting immature behavior. That is, younger nonreferred children and referred children, particularly children with referral problems of immature, distractible behavior in school, had been rated (in 30 second segments) at the highly positive end of the evaluative dimension. If our interpretation of this behavior as immature has been accurate, the observed decrease in positive extremes in children of the Information Feedback group may reflect a more mature behavior pattern and a decrease in "clowning" or "silly" behavior. In part, children's behavior in the initial interaction had been directed "at" the cameras or presumed observers, and the apparent decrease in these behaviors for the children who had the opportunity to see themselves in this way is noteworthy. It suggests a self-chosen and self-imposed behavioral change.

The two parallel sets of changes which were characteristic of Information Feedback families (decreased negative extremes for father and decreased positive extremes for children) were highly correlated ($r = +.96$; $p <$ .01).* The more the father reduced the intensity of his disapproval, the more the child reduced his age-inappropriate "clowning around."

* Using positive peak and negative peak for combined free interaction and problem definition time period.

The other two variables (father directing and father talking) revealed no group differences in change patterns (F Group × Time = .05 for directing; F Group × Time = .41 for talking). All groups of fathers increased in the directiveness of their behavior (F Time = 45.42; $df = 1,5; p < .001$), and there was no change in the amount they talked (F Time = 0.52). Such increased directing behavior by the fathers may reflect an increased effort to elicit desired behavior from their children.

CHANGES IN FAMILY ADJECTIVE RATINGS

Because of the reduced number of cases for which we had complete original and follow-up ratings, the following data again are presented as only indicative of hypothesized changes. They follow consistent themes of the study: the importance of the father-child interaction, and the greater differentiation in the role of the father, as compared to the mother, under different measurement and treatment conditions.

For formal analyses utilizing proportional numbers of cases, we had 10 complete sets of original and follow-up adjective ratings for feedback families, and 10 combined "other" (Parent Counseling and Child Therapy) cases. For each relationship (e.g., father rating mother), a separate Group (feedback versus other) × Time (original versus second follow-up) was computed for the Negative Social Impact factor scores. Significant Group × Time interactions were obtained only for fathers and children. Table 1 indicates two findings for father: (1) A Group × Time effect ($p < .01$) reflects the finding that Information Feedback fathers rated their children more positively after feedback than before. Fathers in the other two groups rated their children as less positive after treatment than before. (2) A Group × Time effect ($p < .05$) reflects the finding that in the Information Feedback group, fathers expected their wives and children to rate them more positively after treatment than before. Fathers in the other two groups expected to be given *less* positive evaluations following treatment.

At follow-up, children in all intervention groups rated both their fathers and themselves more highly (Time effect, $p < .05$) than before treatment. As compared to children in other interventions, Information Feedback youngsters expected to be rated more favorably by the mother at follow-up than before (Group × Time, $p < .05$). However, ratings made by mothers did not change significantly over time, as a result of either feedback or other interventions.

Our hypothesis at this time is that feedback had a significant effect in increasing the father's self-confidence. As noted before, fathers seemed to appear surprised and pleased with their observed interaction with their family and seemed to take a stronger, more assertive stance thereafter. In conjunction with this change it would appear that fathers' increased security enabled

Table 1. Family Adjective Rating Scale—Pre-Post Changes in Information Feedback Versus Other Interventions

	Fa		Mo		Ch	
	IF	Other	IF	Other	IF	Other
Mo	5.21 5.34	4.09 4.55	4.73 5.18	4.92 5.09	5.80 5.98	5.13 5.42
Fa	5.07 5.15	4.98 4.98	5.01 5.16	5.16 4.74	5.51 5.89 T *	4.51 5.25
Ch	3.82 4.25 G × T **	4.60 3.65	4.18 4.52	4.38 4.27	4.72 5.09 T *	4.45 5.20
How Mo will rate	4.42 4.90 G × T **	4.46 4.11			3.72 5.02 G × T **	5.01 4.92
How Fa will rate			4.76 4.99	4.53 4.74	4.99 5.09	4.47 4.87
How Ch will rate	4.94 5.63 G × T **	4.31 4.14	4.66 4.98	4.74 4.70		

them to respond more actively and positively to the child (more like NR fathers). This attention was substantially associated with a decrease in the child's immature behavior. In turn, this change seems associated with improved school grades and decreased problem behavior on the playground. Concomitantly, the fathers' improved self-perception seemed accompanied by the mothers' lowered evaluation of their own effectiveness within the family (TV ratings). This would leave them possibly more willing and able to support their husbands in some of their leadership functions. To whatever extent this occurred, the competition and conflict between parents would decrease and each parent might gradually assume more consistent, culturally role-appropriate behaviors, again providing a source of benefit for the child.

CHAPTER 11

Retrospect and Conclusions

We are reporting findings from endeavors that have spanned almost a decade and involved the intensive collaboration of large groups of people. We have gathered more data than we can currently organize, assimilate, and communicate. Our findings seem important to report but objective evaluation is, of course, impossible for us to achieve. Selective emphases in findings and interpretations are evident in this report, despite our persistent efforts to stay as close as possible to all data. The perspective that would enable us to identify limitations and implications of our work can only be approximated at this time. Certain problems, however, are immediately obvious.

LIMITATIONS, QUALIFICATIONS, AND "WRONG TURNS IN THE MAZE"

1. The small number of girls in our sample precludes any inferences about sex differences, even though trends for girls were generally similar to those obtained for boys. Samples of Hi and Lo SEL families were also small. Generalization from the SEL effects reported must therefore be applied with caution. Moreover, since most Lo SEL cases were black, SEL and race were confounded in this group, again further limiting possible generalizations. Finally, because of the prevalence of broken homes within the referred sample, the number of fathers was reduced markedly in some comparisons; this constitutes yet another restriction upon the generalizability of our results.

2. The decision to omit the Family Adjective Rating Scale, Parent Behavior Inventory, and Communication Task for half the Child Therapy and Parent Counseling families seemed initially appropriate in terms of requirements for the treatment comparisons. Since the results of responding to these instruments were expected to exert some change effect on Information Feedback families, it seemed wise to control for possible effect on treatment outcomes for families in the other intervention groups who took these measures (without feedback). The design niceties represented in this attempt

were almost certainly not commensurate with the value of the family data that was lost, especially since no clear-cut instrument effect appeared in the Parent Counseling and Child Therapy results.

3. Several changes were made during the data gathering processes, for example, in the number of appointments in treatment formats (Chapter 7) and in the administrations of the adjective scales (see Appendix A, p. 241). Though all changes represented improvements in procedure and do not appear to have altered results significantly, it would obviously have been preferable to have followed completely uniform procedures throughout.

4. An early goal was to evaluate the family's behavior in its natural setting, the home, in relation to the behavior observed in the clinic. Observations during home visits to Information Feedback families were planned to collect material for feedback sessions as well as to provide tentative base lines for evaluating family interactions recorded in the clinic. Observation forms (including adjective ratings) were developed for two project workers to complete, independently, after a joint visit in the family home. In numerous pilot visits to pre-project families, however, we ran into two formidable difficulies. (a) Individual families varied widely in the way they structured our visit. Interfamilial comparisons of mother-child contact were not possible, for example, when one mother stayed in the kitchen, insisting on preparing refreshments for family and visitors, whereas another sat on the edge of her chair in the living room, directing the child's every move. (b) Another hindrance to obtaining reliable data in the home was the fact that within each visit the two project members had different experiences. For example, in one home a child was eager to show one consultant the model collection housed in his bedroom while the second consultant was kept in the living room attending to the father's diatribe against the current schoolteacher.

Though it would have been relatively easy to ask families to follow a structured format of interactions during the visit, this would have automatically assumed a role of authority and behavioral control for the visitors. This was diametrically opposed to the basic philosophy of the project and, even more specifically, to the critical objective of the visit: to obtain, in situ, more naturalistically based data than could be obtained in the clinic. Since such individual variations occurred with great regularity we reluctantly decided to observe our project families informally in unstructured visits and hope to develop methods of converting such opportunities into data in some future study. Most consultants did relate impressions that the interactions in the clinic were very similar to behavior in the home, and that the experience of having outsiders visit the home apparently facilitated the development of an objective stance in many families: they seemed to begin considering how their behavior was coming across to someone looking in from the outside—

a basic goal of the approach. But these are impressions which cannot be documented at this time. The time and effort involved in the home visits enriched our personal and clinical understanding of family life in a wide range of physical and sociocultural settings, but added little to our formal project data.

There were two other instances of nonsignificant data in our project. Pediatric examinations of first year children and responses to a Family Value Questionnaire both failed to indicate significant trends and so have not been intensively analyzed.

5. The focus of most of this study was on specific, overt behaviors of individuals, sometimes in sequential segments which were parts of interpersonal exchanges. This strategy seems to have yielded consistent patterns across different sets of data, as has been described. In the analyses many clues were obtained about the larger interactional patterns and processes. So far, however, our formal analyses have not dealt with more complex units of interpersonal interactions.

6. The use of evaluation, directiveness, and activity as major dimensions of behavior seems to have worked well in providing a unifying framework for our family findings. As indicated in the preceding paragraph, however, analyses were limited to the behavior of individuals, so even the descriptive use of the interpersonal dimensions was based on incomplete (i.e., not truly interpersonal) data.

7. In our studies of conflicting evaluative components in parental messages recorded on videotapes, there are basic questions which require further investigation. For instance, messages may be addressed simultaneously to more than one receiver. This involves not only the probability that some message components may be "sweetened" for the benefit of presumed observers, but also such possibilities as that a mother's positive verbal message to a child may be accompanied by a negative nonverbal component, signaled in one flashing glance directed toward someone else in the room. The analysis of verbal and nonverbal behavior via videotape recording is a challenging new area of research. The problems inherent in recording completely *natural* behavior without violation of privacy and confidentiality remains to be resolved. With time we would hope that such recording may become less threatening, and so less constraining.

8. Adjective scales used as indicators of interpersonal perception apparently picked up significant nuances within family units (FARS, Chapter 3). We have not yet assessed the effect of our use of standard definitions for the adjectives. These were included in the hope that greater commonality of meanings held for the adjectives during the rating process would reduce a major source of variability in ratings. The procedure is believed to have

been effective in this regard, but further work is needed to evaluate the exact contribution of this presumed refinement.

9. In planning the selection of school observers to rate children's behavior we had hoped to include both men and women, as well as raters from all socioeconomic levels. Because of the part-time nature of the work this was possible only if we had used a much older group of potential observers, an alternative which we rejected. Our school raters therefore were made up of middle-class women who were probably not too different from the teachers themselves (except in terms of specific educational and vocational backgrounds).

10. Probably the greatest weakness of our overall efforts was in our work in the schools. The cost in time and money of training observers and getting them accepted in the school setting was very great indeed. It is obvious that our payoff in terms of the data obtained was sometimes disappointing. Although all findings were in expected directions, and usually at acceptable levels of significance, many were by and large so general as to do little except validate commonsense predictions. Although this is in itself a worthwhile methodological goal to achieve, we of course had hoped for greater specificity in many school findings.

We believe that the weakness of the school data is due to three major factors. (1) The first is that in gaining administrators' acceptance of our observers in the school, we were obliged to focus on the child, excluding observations of teacher behaviors. Teacher behavior patterns, in conjunction with parental behaviors described previously, probably contributed significantly to the child's specific response at school. It seems likely that until we can get information on teacher-child interactions (perhaps in the form of recordings of complete interactions in the school setting which are comparable to our family video recordings) we will not be able to specify detailed relationships between child behavior and its interpersonal context at school. We believe that, like parents, most teachers want to assist children in learning and maturing. But we also suspect that many teachers have little more expertise than other adults in recognizing the characteristics of their verbal and nonverbal behavior that directly (or in conflictual combination with parental behavior) pose difficulty, provocation, or distress for some of the children they teach. (2) Results from the school settings were also constrained by the situational settings in which observations could be made. The highly structured didactic process which prevailed in most classrooms often permitted few behavioral opportunities for the children being observed. In the end, these classroom data were of little value. (3) On the playground, arrangements in different schools varied widely, so that behaviors were influenced greatly by situational variability. In sum, though we were glad to have the opportunity to observe the children as they "naturally" acted in an everyday setting, we suffered from the usual handicaps in obtaining reliable data from naturalistic settings.

There are doubtless other, and possibly more critical, limitations in our work than those we have recognized so far, but the foregoing serve as sharp reminders of our problems and of the restrictions on the generalizability of our findings.

Despite the difficulties encountered in our work, however, we view our results as generally making good sense. They support and amplify much of the major research in parent-child, family, school, treatment, and socioeconomic level areas. And they provide new data that detail meaningful interconnections for earlier findings within these different areas.

IMPLICATIONS

Family and School Findings

The differences in daily experiences with adults found for nonreferred as compared to referred children provide some substantiation for our original hypothesis that the child's ongoing interpersonal environment is critical for his social effectiveness, at least as manifested in the school setting.

Methodologically, the information derived from our four sets of family data seems useful in providing comparisons between expressed attitudes and observed behavior. A comparison of the findings from the four sources shows that the more detailed, specific, and complete the information recorded (e.g., the nonverbal as well as verbal data available for repeated review in videotapes of total family interaction), the more useful it is in adding to our understanding of interpersonal behavior. This emphasis on concrete, specific, current, behavioral data was conceptually basic to the Information Feedback intervention.

The various findings demonstrate the effects on children's home and school behavior that are related to differing parental relationships, roles, and patterns. Within the family, we note that the specific characteristics identified are consistent with the description of family role dynamics offered years ago by Parson and Bales. In this formulation mothers were seen as exercising largely expressive roles associated with the management of interpersonal and emotional affairs of the family, whereas fathers' roles were identified more with instrumental tasks, like providing economic support and managing major problem-solving tasks in the family. These authors interpret the development of family-role behavior within a largely psychoanalytic framework. We share their belief that such psychodynamic variables are important bases of behavior. But we believe that interpersonal behaviors are also profoundly and continuously influenced by situational and social forces. When seen from the perspective of those ongoing environmental influences, any particular form of family organization characteristic of present or past cultures may not be an inevitable characteristic of "human nature." This point may be illustrated by briefly reviewing some of our relevant results and the implications which we draw from them.

In our nonreferred families, the complementary role relationships between parents that seemed associated with children's effective behavior at school were specified in some detail. Each parent had mutually recognized areas of responsibility; each was trusted and supported by the spouse in his own role-appropriate areas; children knew and accepted the differential parental authority; at this age they did not seriously question or challenge parental roles or responsibilities.

Beyond this, however, our findings indicate that the *active involvement of the father in the child's life seemed an essential ingredient for effective adaptation at home and at school.* When, as often happened in our referred families, the mother continued to play the predominant parental role during these years, there was an increased probability that the child would have difficulty in his interpersonal adjustment.

In our referred families there was much evidence that parenthood was an onerous responsibility for which people felt ill-equipped. Similarly the personal relations between marital partners were apparently joyless and distrustful. The same theme of meager, unsatisfying interpersonal relationships was reported in relation to their adult communities. Within such a consistent context of interpersonal inadequacy it would be remarkable indeed if children were to emerge with good personal and social skills and competencies. *The consistency of these differential patterns emphasizes the need for means to be developed whereby people can improve their interpersonal competence and comfort, both for their own fulfilment and to increase the potential for their children's optimal development.*

In realistic terms we found that the psychological adequacy of adults could not be viewed separately from the economic and social pressures that beset them (socioeconomic level variations, single-parent conditions, and the like). Our environmental emphasis, in fact, turned out to be applicable at three levels of generality, for both adults and children: (1) pressures related to broad socioeconomic and sociocultural differences and deficits; (2) specific demands associated with failure to fit easily into current social role patterns and cultural expectations; (3) stresses deriving from immediate interpersonal contexts in daily life. Though we posit no simple causal mechanisms, our data identify relationships of adaptive versus maladaptive behavior with each of these sources of potential difficulty, and in the myriad interconnections between them.

1. SEL: for adults the clearest example of the first of these potential hazards is the pressure associated with Lo SEL and the high probability of family disruption that often seems to attend it. Increased economic and social demands impinged on the Lo SEL R mother, for example, while her personal and interpersonal resources were simultaneously restricted. (That SEL effects are not simple, however, must be kept in mind: Lo SEL NR families reflected no more familial disruption than control families at other levels.) For Lo SEL fathers the well-known difficulties of becoming assimilated into the larger social and economic community were exemplified clearly. For Lo SEL children, there were differences in cultural backgrounds and deficits in the kinds of past experiences which interfered with adaptation to the task oriented classroom behavior expected by their (usually) middle-class teachers. In spite of obvious efforts on the part of school personnel to allow for the sources of these differences, discrepancies remained which were reflected in negative teacher evaluations of the Lo SEL children, both referred and nonreferred.

The fact that our Lo SEL group was made up entirely of minority families, most of them black, makes it impossible to know whether the difficulties exhibited in these instances were related to economic deficiencies, racial problems (e.g., discrimination in terms of restricted education, mobility, and jobs) or some combination of both. In any case our findings are consonant with other research and highlight serious social problems that demand the attention and change efforts of our political and social institutions: Lo SEL children need the experience of fitting comfortably and effectively into a congruent school environment.

Similar SEL effects show up in different types of pressure for children at other SEL's. Mid SEL R children seemed predisposed, as a group, to become inhibited in their interactions, whereas the aggressive interpersonal style of the Hi SEL R pupils was regarded in highly negative terms by their teachers. *Each of these SEL effects needs investigation and delineation as a necessary step toward a realistic assessment of the expectations for children's behavior in school, the appropriateness of such expectations, and the development of effective means of helping children cope with such expectations. The interpersonal mechanisms through which such SEL effects are mediated in the school situation require exploration and specification since they seem likely to be significant sources of some of the interpersonal difficulties children experience.*

2. Social expectations: this second set of problems was apparent in all

four measures of familial behavior and was exemplified most clearly by the role relationships of some referred fathers and mothers. This pattern seemed to represent a reversal of culturally defined paternal and maternal roles. For many of the parents in our referred group, such stereotypes for male and female roles seemed to be a source of considerable discomfort and dissatisfaction (though there were certainly others). Some of the mothers appeared to be sitting on the sidelines, chafing with unused energy, feeling very critical of their husbands and implying that they could be more effective in the instrumental role than their husbands were. (Observers were sometimes inclined to agree that they indeed might.) By the same token, referred fathers often seemed to feel that inordinate amounts of responsibility were foisted on them, that familial demands and expectations were more than they could meet. Thus role responsibilities often seemed very poor fits to individual personalities and seemed therefore relatively unattainable.

From this point of view, trends in today's society which permit greater individual choice in the ways role responsibilities can be allocated and shared between parental partners would seem a potentially constructive development. As the areas of overlap in terms of men's and women's experience increase we might expect a broadened basis for mutual understanding and interpersonal accommodation. Though our findings have emphasized the necessity for stable interrelated roles on the part of adults in the child's life, the *complementarity* of roles would seem, speculatively, more important than the *content* of role assignments. Current role changes seem to involve the definition of role behaviors on bases other than biologically determined sex functions. This follows quite naturally from the fact that modern technology has already made some sex-based roles seem outdated (e.g., the inadequate challenge many women find when they are restricted to the role of "wife and mother," or the excessive pressure experienced by some men when they feel they must pursue stereotyped "masculine" goals to points that far exceed their personal proclivities or capacities). From this point of view our data may be interpreted to indicate that *(a)* a stable, mutually satisfactory and complementary arrangement is needed which *(b)* has substantial acceptance on the larger social scene: children's mastery of their environment seems to be facilitated if roles learned in the home are consonant with the expectations of the larger world outside.

If the culture assimilates these more varied and flexible role patterns, individualized arrangements within a parental unit would be less unusual and should constitute less of a hazard for the child when he seeks to apply in the external world the role perceptions he learned at home.

But cultural changes usually take time to evolve and to become consolidated within a society. The probability seems great that in the intervening years, while newer role models are fluctuating and even contradictory in pattern and social value, many children may experience intensified difficulty in acquiring personal security and interpersonal skills. The sense of individual identity, the role definitions, and the expectations that seem necessary for effective interpersonal functioning may well be difficult for some children to achieve when the very goals of socialization (e.g., "masculine" identity) are in flux. The hope for the interim is that the adults' increased sense of personal freedom and fulfillment will be great enough to offset some of the difficulties their idiosyncratic role patterns may constitute for their children.

A second hopeful indication for children's welfare is the vastly augmented individual choice about having children in the first place. Though very little is known about the motivation and meanings related to having children, there is overwhelming evidence for the deleterious effects of having (or being) an unwanted child. As the incidence of such undesired "burdens" declines, opportunities should increase for adults to feel adequate in their parental roles, along social, economic, and psychological dimensions. As long as people have only the children they want and feel able to look after, they may be able to enjoy their interactions with them more, and find the relationship a more pleasurable experience. Since children no longer represent any potential economic gain (indeed, quite the contrary), they must apparently be viewed as potential sources of *psychological* gain by their parents. Both their initial dependency and their unfolding patterns of competence and autonomy must somehow imply some potential for emotional gratification for their parents. This at least seemed the way in which children were regarded and valued by the control in comparison to referred parents in the present study.

3. The immediate interpersonal environment: the third source of environmental pressure is the one toward which our work was basically directed, the identification of the potentially noxious consequences for a child that inhere in his daily interactions with parents and teachers. A number of these have been delineated, in varying degrees of specificity and detail. We also attempted to demonstrate that adults' attention to these interpersonal phenomena can be stimulated, such that new information will be sought and utilized by them in ways that improve the quality of the child's daily social experiences. The techniques and goals of Information Feedback are of course only one way of approaching the general goal of increasing interpersonal comfort and competence.

Treatment Results

Our treatment comparisons emphasized the need for a range of interventions for children's developmental difficulties. These apparently will be most effective if they focus on the significant adults who deal with the child, and if they permit appropriate matching between the intervention and certain characteristics of these parents and teachers. These involve variation in socioeconomic level and perhaps some psychological characteristics such as predilections for relatively autonomous or dependent relationships. In this context the major contribution of procedures such as those in Information Feedback is the facilitation of people's use of their general problem-solving capacities in interpersonal areas.

Secondly, the results suggest that long-term impact on gross indicators of behavior (grades) can be obtained by a procedure which seeks to minimize the introduction of new values, standards, or indeed any stipulation for how people should behave. Ideally, Information Feedback should do nothing except provide techniques through which people examine their behavior, discover questions, and experiment with changes they desire. Thus when a parent or teacher is concerned about a child, his first step is to survey behavior in order to get more information about the child's interactions with the significant adults in his life. A specific, current scanning of the antecedents and consequences of these interactions for the child will usually provide a new recognition of (a) what the adult does or can do that will elicit a different response from the child and (b) how the child's behavior affects the adult.

Except for assuming that it is desirable to assist people to increase their range of information about themselves and each other, there are no necessary assumptions in Information Feedback about desirable or "healthy" ways in which people should act toward each other. Minimizing professional interference in people's lives is, for us, an important value, so that we are encouraged by evidence that our procedures are at least as facilitative of behavior change as are more directive interventions.

A second important consequence of our work with this approach is its implication for further work with schools and others in the community. As we consult with community members, our stance becomes explicitly that of a particular type of catalyst-facilitator. We focus attention on participants' efforts to gather information about themselves and others in the environment. We assist in devising techniques for obtaining and displaying information, but we offer little with respect to its meaning or use. We take this position not especially on moral grounds, but because we are convinced that solutions reached on the basis of outsiders' meanings or values will be short-lived and ineffective. Since no persons, and especially no groups, have identical value systems, we expect that the ultimately useful solutions are those that for an individual are self-selected, and for a group are determined by whatever internal consensus its members can hammer out.

In summary, our goal is to enable individuals to broaden the range, increase the accuracy, and verify for themselves the validity of their own perceptions, communications, and interpersonal behaviors. This seems at least a valid alternative to other types of behavior change approaches.

Development and Standardization
of Instruments

SOCIOECONOMIC LEVEL CLASSIFICATION OF FAMILIES
AND SCHOOLS

The identification of ten schools representing the socioeconomic range of the West Los Angeles District was accomplished with the help of district administrators of the Los Angeles City Schools. Additionally, census tract information collected by the UCLA Department of Sociology provided data on housing, income, education, and employment. This specified the predominant socioeconomic level of the population served by each school. Cases referred from any one school, and from schools at the same SEL, were remarkably similar with respect to parents' occupation and education, as well as family housing characteristics.

Socioeconomic level for individual families was determined by the socioeconomic level of the school. To check the accuracy of this index, half of the sample was also rated by the Hollingshead five point method (Hollingshead, 1958), but combining the two top levels and the two bottom levels to yield a three point scale. The two methods yielded identical classifications in all but two cases. On this basis the three point classification provided by school area designation seemed sufficient. Use of this relatively rough categorization (high, middle, low) was dictated by sample size. The usual five point classification would have yielded too small an N for meaningful statistical analysis, especially when each level was subdivided in terms of referred, nonreferred, or referral category subgroups.

INDEX OF FUNCTIONAL VERBAL FACILITY

Families in the project participated in complex tasks which required that verbal instructions be understood and followed. It was important to guard against the possibility that differences in task performance might be related more to verbal facility than to group differences (e.g., whether referred or nonreferred). We therefore tried to obtain verbal IQ estimates for all participants. Many of the referred children had received either a Binet or WISC at school, but no uniform reference scale was initially available for all project children. There was equal need for a measure of intellectual functioning for the parents, though we did not have access to enough parental time to do a thorough individual assessment. The wide range of socioeconomic levels in the sample precluded using a measure emphasizing abstract verbal skills or paper and pencil tests, so the Ammons' Full Range Picture-Vocabulary Test (FRPV) was finally chosen (Ammons and Huth, 1949). This seemed a fairly reliable and valid rough screening instrument with a high correlation with more standard measures of intelligence (e.g., Dickinson, Neubert, & McDermott, 1968). When we later compared the FRPV IQ with any IQ score available from the schools, the FRPV IQ index was highly correlated with WISC and Binet scores but was consistently higher than either. Parents appeared to achieve less inflated scores on this task than did children, through no adult comparison scores on other tests were available for the parents.

The FRPV was used as only a rough screening for functional verbal facility relevant to the project tasks. The test was administered individually to parents and target children during either their first or second visit to the clinic. Because we were constantly faced with time priorities (when a family arrived late, for example) we chose, when necessary, to omit the FRPV rather than other data. IQ data were obtained from 40 referred fathers, 52 referred mothers, and 81 referred childen. Nonreferred data included 26 fathers, 28 mothers, and all 29 children.

GRADES

Children's school grades, A through F, were converted into numerical values: A = 4, B = 3, C = 2, D = 1, and F = 0. Grades for each child were collected for three semesters prior to intake and at least three semesters after intake. Separate Kaiser Varimax factor analyses of grade scores at different grade levels failed to yield completely consistent orthogonally rotated factor structures. Music and art, physical education (PE), and conduct evaluations (the child's effort, work habits, and citizenship) almost always fell into three separate factors in three or more replications. Academic grades usually constituted a separate factor group but in several analyses some academic grades were distributed among the other three factors. In the end it seemed most representative of analyses made over all grade levels to put academic grades (reading, spoken and written English, handwriting, spelling, arithmetic, geography, history, civics, and science) into one grouping. We therefore had four separate grade groupings for each child: his scores for music-art, physical education, conduct, and academic subjects. A child's score in any group was the average of his grades in the different subject areas included in that group. In addition, we used an overall index of a child's performance at a given time by averaging all his grades in all graded areas. The total score is most heavily weighted by grades in the academic area since there are more of them. This index was used as the major outcome measure: changes in the child's overall adaptation at school over time and treatments.

REFERRAL CATEGORY CLASSIFICATIONS

To examine the quantitative relation between types of referral problems and our various process and outcome measures, we developed a method for classifying each child's problem and indicating its severity. As with all categories and measures, we tried to base our indices as closely as possible on children's overt behaviors. The description of the child's difficulties on the school referral form served as the basis for classification. The referral statement was broken into references to each problem behavior mentioned (e.g., "is restless," "often fights with other children"). The number of such items in referral statements ranged from 1 through 15. Statements pertaining to academic problems, which occurred in 81% of the cases, were excluded from this analysis.

Three judges from the project staff independently sorted all items into individually determined categories, with prior agreement to use no more than five divisions. Four common groupings emerged in each of the three independent sortings: (1) *Direct Aggression* (Ag) included mention of overt, physically aggressive, or verbally hostile behavior. (2) *Hyperactivity* (Hy) involved social difficulties including restlessness, talking out in class, and other high activity forms of social deviance which did not include direct personal attack (aggression); it also included its inevitable correlate, poor peer relationships. (3) *Social Withdrawal* (SW) included fearfulness and limited social interactions. Somatic symptoms, though not overt behaviors, typically appeared in conjunction with these indications of interpersonal inhibition, and so were subsumed in this classification. (4) *Attention Control* (AC) included failure to follow directions, the need for continuous supervision, immature behavior, laziness, poor work habits, and inability to concentrate.

Each statement on a child referral form was categorized and given a severity rating. The sum of the entries in each problem category was computed, with the highest of the four values determining the child's predominant classification.

The severity scores were determined in the following way. In most cases, more than one item in a statement referred to behaviors falling within the same category. For example, "has trouble paying attention," "is lazy," and "can't concentrate" all relate to attention control. Each item was judged as an independent statement and was given a score ranging from 1 (minimal severity) to 7 (maximum severity). Degree of severity was judged in terms of commonly accepted word meanings and the use of modifiers indicating intensity or frequency. A simple behavior quality without indication of either frequency or intensity was placed at the middle of the scale: thus "restless" (Hy), "aggressive" (Ag), "avoids others" (SW), or "lazy" (AC), were all given values of four on their relevant scales. Values were increased or decreased in terms of specifications of either frequency or intensity. For example, when these words were preceded with modifiers indicating low intensity ("seems a little shy"), the scale value of an item was decreased. Similar variations in intensity or frequency could be indicated by the specificity or generality of the terms in which the behavior was described. Thus "hyperactive" alone was considered to refer to a generalized behavior pattern and given a relatively high score of five, as compared with "moves around in class" which was rated as two. Three judges agreed on the category classification of statements in 87% of sortings and agreed on the scale placement of items within a category within a range of three scale points in 71% of the cases. Disagreement was resolved by obtaining consensus among the three judges.

Every child was given a severity score for each category, with each score computed according to a formula developed for this purpose $[(\Sigma X^2 + N\Sigma X)/(\Sigma X + N)]$. In this formula X refers to the scale value of an item classified in a given category and N is the number of items within this category mentioned for the child by the referring school staff. This formula not only takes heavy account of the modal value of items but also considers both the number of statements and their scale value. It seemed that if a teacher had a great deal to say about a child, this probably reflected more concern about him than when she said very little. However, the frequent mention of relatively slight problems should carry less weight than a single mention of more severe problems. The formula takes these requirements into account. The referral statement regarding any particular child did not usually include all four categories, so that most subjects have zero in one or more categories. This clustering of a large number of zeros in each category produced high variance which was minimized by subjecting all subject category scores to a $(X + 1)^{1/2}$ transformation.

Severity scores within categories ranged between 0 and 11.52 when all referral statements had been categorized according to this system. An example of a high severity score on aggressiveness (9.51) for a Hi SEL 11 year old boy is based on these comments on the referral form: "is extremely belligerent when things don't go his way; spends much of his time anticipating problems which hinders his learning processes; he has a very difficult time admitting that he is wrong or that he has made a mistake; very poor peer relations in the classroom and on the yard; needs to learn how to relate to people properly and accept criticism; he will hit other students if he doesn't like something they have said or done; extremely sensitive; takes things personally; must learn to display self-control and be responsible for his own action."

An example of a case with low severity (2.00) is a 12 year old boy in the Attention Control category whose teacher attributed his inability to be still in class entirely to frustration because of his inability to learn. The referral statement read: "because he cannot be successful in his work (he has dyslexia, is a nonreader) he draws frequently, chatters, and plays with objects in his desk."

This classification scheme, it is emphasized, grows out of perception of the child's behavior at school and so might well deviate somewhat from other categorizations. Becker et. al., (1959), Peterson (1961), and Quay and Quay (1963) report that much of the systematic variance associated with maladaptive behavior at this age can be accounted for by two orthogonal dimensions, aggression or conduct-deviant behavior and withdrawn or personality-deviant behavior. As will become clearer in the light of material to be presented, our categories I and II, Aggressiveness and Hyperactivity, are quite similar to their conduct-deviant dimension, and our III and IV, Social Withdrawal and Attention Control, seem to represent behavioral correlates of personality factors. Thus there seems to be considerable overlap in these classification systems of children's behavior.

THE ADJECTIVE RATING SCALE

Development

The Adjective Rating Scale was developed over a 2 year period with pilot testing of over 350 individuals, including college students and sets of parents and their elementary-school aged children. The adjectives were selected on three bases: (1) they must be comprehensible to most third grade children and to adults with little schooling; (2) they should refer to common, overt attributes or behaviors identifiable with minimal ambiguity; and (3) they should have relevance for interpersonal functioning. We finally selected a set of 20 adjectives which satisfied the above criteria: *active, calm, clear,* confident, dependable, friendly,* happy, patient,* smart, controlling,* afraid,* phony,* angry,* bad, bored,* lazy, mean, nagging, rude,* selfish.*

The general procedure was to give each rater (parent, child, teacher, or project observer) a denotative definition for each adjective, emphasizing that he was to use this, and *only* this, meaning of the word. The definitions were obtained from fourth, fifth, and sixth grade students in a ghetto school outside the project area and resulted in simple succinct statements (e.g., "friendly" means liking people and being nice to them). Since these words were to be used by many people and in many contexts, we wanted to specify their meanings very concretely to increase the uniformity of the measuring unit and thus improve both reliability and validity of the scales.

In addition to specifying denotative definitions for each word, we attempted to assess the range of affective meanings the adjectives had for each user. To do this, we asked each rater to rate each *adjective* on a five point semantic differential scale, (Osgood, Suci, & Tannenbaum, 1957), on the following dimensions: "good-bad" for evaluation, "fast-slow" for activity, and "hot-cold" and "strong-weak" for potency. The variance of these ratings was so small as to indicate almost universal agreement among subjects as to the meaning of these words. We therefore assumed that the adjectives constituted a fairly stable frame of reference for the individual raters.

Pilot testing was done to establish test-retest reliability for different methods of administration, and to check the stability of the factor-structure when used by different kinds of raters in different situations. The test-retest reliability (2 week interval) for college age adults ranged from .53 to .83 with a median of .67. However, for children, the median test-retest reliability coefficient was only .45. This low reliability is in line with results reported by others, but requires that results of children's ratings be interpreted with much caution.

Ten factor analyses were made on adjective ratings of children viewed in different contexts (playground, classroom, clinic, home) by a variety of raters (teachers, independent raters, parents). Samples used in the factor analyses included ratings of random, referred, and normal control children with sample sizes ranging from 79 to 118. Two factors consistently emerged in all analyses: a Negative Social Impact factor (IB) which included the adjectives *"angry"* (high), *"patient"* (low), *"phony"* (high), and *"rude"* (high); and a Positive Social Impact or interpersonal adaptivity factor (IIB) which included the adjectives *"controlling"* (high), *"bored"* (low),

---

*The asterisks indicate the subset of 10 adjectives which were used throughout the project when ongoing interpersonal behavior was being judged.

"active" (high), and *"friendly"* (high). Any adjectives to be retained in a factor had to have a factor loading of .40 or higher in at least two out of three settings (home, school, clinic) in which these independent ratings were made. One adjective, "controlling," had high loadings on both factors (negative and positive impact). It was placed on the positive scale because it most consistently emerged on this factor across all sets of ratings. Ratings were analyzed and are presented in terms of these two factors throughout this volume. "Afraid" usually loaded highly as a residual factor; therefore it was dropped from all analyses.

Pilot Studies Using the Adjective Rating Scale

During this development, this scale was examined by administering it to several populations, two of which are reported here. One consisted of college students who varied in the level of self-described anxiety. The second consisted of families of children enrolled in a special school for children with learning disabilities.

COLLEGE STUDENTS

Sixty-five male and 62 female undergraduates participating as part of an introductory course requirement were given the following instruments: (1) a 20-adjective scale (from which the 10-adjective list was later derived) with each subject rating the following concepts: the average person of his age and sex, himself, his father, his mother, the general atmosphere of his home and how he would like to be, that is, his ideal self; (2) the Semantic Differential which included his rating of each adjective as a concept (e.g., "friendly") on a seven point good-bad scale; (3) the 20-item version of the manifest anxiety scale (Howe & Silverstein, 1960); (4) a brief questionnaire in which each person was asked to rate the extent to which he felt that he understood each of his parents and, in turn, felt understood by them.

For purposes of this study, the adjective rating on each concept was multiplied by the person's rating of the *adjective* on the good-bad semantic differential scale. Thus if a person rated the word "friendly" as 6 on the semantic differential, and rated his mother as 5 on friendly his score would be 30. We then took the square root of this score and added all the other scores for each of the adjectives rated on this concept so as to obtain a total weighted score.

To obtain a rough index of self-described psychological effectiveness, we divided the distribution of manifest anxiety scale scores into quartiles, quartile one representing lowest anxiety scores and quartile four the highest. Subjects were tested in groups of 30–35 subjects.

The results of the adjective rating scale were analyzed by Anxiety Level

$\times$ Sex $\times$ Concept analysis of variance. The main anxiety effect was significant with an $F = 3.26$, $df = 3,120$, $p < .05$. The results indicated that highly anxious subjects, especially those in the fourth quartile, are different from those of low anxious subjects, especially those in the first and second quartile, on ratings of self, father, and the atmosphere of the home. There were no differences in ratings of the mother, the average person, or the ideal self. On the questionnaire data, an Anxiety Level $\times$ Questionnaire Scale analysis of variance yielded $F = 3.93$, $df = 3,124$, $p < .01$, indicating that the more anxious subjects felt less well understood by their parents and, in turn, felt that they understood their parents less well than did the subjects with less anxiety. Other results obtained for this pilot group were typical of those obtained with other pilot groups on whom we pretested the adjective rating scale. It is of some interest that these initial ratings by young adults prefigured the differences in the evaluations of father and mother which were found so consistently throughout this study.

STUDIES WITH FAMILIES

Through the cooperation of the UCLA Fernald School staff, we were able to study the families of children enrolled in summer school. These children were of at least average intelligence but had been manifesting serious learning problems in their regular school. There were 65 boys who ranged in age from 8 to 13. Most of the families were from middle and upper-middle socioeconomic levels.

The parents were first given the Semantic Differential scale, as described above, followed by the Adjective Rating Scale on which they rated the following concepts in turn: myself, my child, how my child will rate me. The parents were then asked to fill out a brief questionnaire providing data on family background including education, family income, type of occupation, and the child's grades in regular school. They made ratings of their relations with the child and of the general home atmosphere. In addition, they rated the child's current anxiety level, reported the frequency and reasons for school conferences during the previous year, and indicated whether or not they felt the child to be in need of psychological help for emotional or behavioral problems. Teachers rated the child's anxiety level, his peer relations, behavior in the classroom, and academic performance. The children were also given the Semantic Differential and Adjective Rating Scale. Especially with the younger children, however, much difficulty was encountered in their understanding of the Semantic Differential (in the preliminary form we were using at that time) and it was therefore abandoned for this pilot investigation. The children also filled out the Sarason General Anxiety Test.

In order to estimate psychological "disturbance" levels in the children, five of the items were selected as criteria in the following ways: anxiety level ratings by parent, teacher, and the child himself (Sarason Anxiety Scale) were counted as indicating "disturbance" for a given case *only* if scored in the top quartile of the sample distribution. The school-parent conference items counted when more than two such conferences had been called by the school during the past year because of the child's emotional and behavioral problems. The fifth item was the parent's statement that the child currently needed psychological help. Any criterion item based on parents' ratings was counted only once, even if both parents agreed. Level of disturbance was determined according to the following arbitrary rules: high disturbance (Hi group)—all five of the above items exceeded criterion levels. Moderate disturbance (M group)—two or three of the five items were beyond the cutoff level. Low disturbance (Lo group)—no more than one item indicated significant anxiety. This procedure classified 18 cases in the Hi group, 36 in the M group, and 28 in the Lo group. The three groups of children did not differ significantly in age or academic performance in summer school. They did differ significantly, ($p < .01$), on teacher grades of conduct, work habits, and cooperation, with the Hi group receiving the worst grades. Since the children's semantic differential ratings were not usable, and the factor analyses for the adjectives had not been conducted at that time, these results were analyzed by dividing the 20 adjectives into 10 which, according to semantic differential ratings on the good-bad scale had positive connotations, and another group of 10 with predominantly negative connotations. The results were analyzed with a Disturbance Level × Sex (mother, father) × Concept analysis of variance, separately for the negative and positive list of words. For the negative list the disturbance level yielded an $F = 8.27$, $df = 2,144$, $p < .01$. There was no main sex effect nor was there a disturbance by sex interaction. There was, however, a strong disturbance by concept interaction ($F = 5.36$, $df = 4,288$, $p < .01$). This was due to the fact that, for both parents, their evaluation of the child was related directly to its categorization in the disturbance categories, with the Hi disturbance children rated as most negative, and the Lo children rated as least negative. There was much less variation in the parents' ratings of themselves or in their expectations of how the child would rate them. The parents of the Hi children expected to be rated more negatively than the parents in the other two groups. On the ratings of self, only the fathers' ratings showed a relation between disturbance category and self-evaluation, in that each Hi father rated himself more negatively than either the Mid or the Lo fathers. The mothers' self-ratings did not vary according to the child's disturbance group. On the positive words there was no significant effect for disturbance category ($F = 2.30$, $df = 2,138$, $p > .05$). Ratings by the children on either negative or positive words did not reach the .05 level.

Again, these early results are in line with the R/NR differences reported for family ratings in Chapter 3. These pilot studies also indicated the necessity for incorporating individual administration of procedures for children at this age level. On the basis of these experiences demonstration materials were worked up and used whenever either children or adults had difficulty in understanding either the concepts or procedures involved in making ratings.

Differences in Year I and Year II

During the first year of data collection we used all twenty adjectives in measuring the perceptions of family members. When we evaluated our activities at the end of the year, we recognized that the family ratings, reflecting general attitudes about *persons,* were less relevant than the perceptions of specific *behaviors* on which our measures throughout the project were focused. There was no way to refer these general ratings to specific behaviors at any particular place and time. We needed to further define and delimit the frame of reference within which family ratings were made.

We therefore reluctantly decided to change the method for the second-year families. After completing the Semantic Differential, the parents and target child in second-year families were asked to rate the behavior which they could recall observing during the "Problem Definition" phase of their interaction, completed a few minutes before. Instructions emphasized that ratings should focus on the behaviors which they remembered as having occurred during that period. We do not assume, of course, that we were able to make a radical change in the set of the raters because they were still rating "people." Hopefully, however, they were doing so in a somewhat more current and behavioral context.

A second change made between Year I and Year II of the data collection was the reduction of the number of adjectives used. The rating process using the original 20-word list for each of six concepts took about an hour's time, and not all of the adjectives seemed equally pertinent to rating of interpersonal behavior. The 10-word subset which was used in school observations and other parts of the study was substituted. The adjectives were *calm, patient, clear, friendly, active, controlling, bored, angry, rude,* and *phony.*

When all of the second-year data had been collected, we studied the differences obtained in the two sets of ratings. The rank order correlation between means of the 10 adjectives common to both applications (e.g., father's ratings of himself in the "global," first-year context as compared with his recall of behaviors in the family interaction, second-year condition) ranged between .66 and .93, with a median of .78. A more important comparison was to examine referred-nonreferred differences between the two applications for each adjective, considering only "self" and "other" ratings.

There were 30 comparisons for each rater (e.g., Fa-Self, Fa-Mo, Fa-Ch for each of the 10 adjectives). Overall, referred-nonreferred differences for global and immediate recall ratings were in the same direction in 85% of the comparisons. Compared to the nonreferred parents, referred parents tended to rate themselves and each other more unfavorably on the immediate recall than on the global ratings (recall R/NR differences were lower than global differences in 72% of the comparisons). The child's ratings were less consistent than the parents' for the two ratings (8 of 30 R/NR differences were reversed), but the overall referred-nonreferred differences were still in the same direction. As children's ratings usually have lower test-retest reliability, this inconsistency is not unexpected.

Since conclusions about referred-nonreferred differences were the same for all comparisons of global and immediate recall applications, the individual ratings were converted into C scores to permit combined statistical treatment for first- and second-year families. The different reference criteria for the two sets of data must be considered in the evaluation of results. For example, the more negative results in the recall (second year) ratings of referred parents would seem reasonably related to their recalling the anxiety attendant upon their first clinic visit and the knowledge of being observed and recorded. This situational effect might be expected to lead to intensified differences between the referred and nonreferred families. In point of fact, however, the videotapes of the interactions being recalled indicate many similarities in the behaviors of the two sets of families under this condition in both years. The statistical significance of the R/NR comparisons, overall, seems clear.

THE PARENT BEHAVIOR INVENTORY

This inventory was developed over a period of 2 years. In this time, approximately 200 sets of parents (from the University of California's Fernald School, the University Elementary School, and poverty-area public schools) were given different versions of the inventory. In most of these preliminary investigations, the questions were administered orally to permit detailed exploration of the comprehensibility of the task and specific items in it. Only those questions were kept which were easily understood by subjects with little education and where the range of scores for at least 50% of responses was greater than two adjacent score points. When we were satisfied that the items were clear, had adequate variance, and that substantial portions of the instrument differentiated between parents of disturbed and nondisturbed children, 95 mothers and 80 fathers drawn from the pilot population filled out a version of the inventory very similar to the final form. Results were factor-analyzed using a Kaiser Varimax rotation. Items which loaded less than .40 on any factor and factors containing less than three items were eliminated. Because of the limitation of the factor analysis programs the inventory had to be factored in three sections. One section contained the items relating primarily to the child's behavior in relation to the parent. Another contained the parent's behavior in relation to the child. The third section covered items describing relations of the parents to each other and the family's relation to the community.

These factor analyses were later replicated with the project sample. At that point, in order to maximize reliability of factors, it was desirable to have a larger number of subjects than was available in the project population. To achieve this, the project sample was supplemented with additional sets of Fernald School and University Elementary School parents, making a total of 95 mothers and 80 fathers for the replication. About four-fifths of the items appeared in the same factors in both sets of factor analyses, so that we can consider the factor structure reported here quite reliable. Items which showed a radical shift in factor structure from one analysis to the other were eliminated. Where an item loaded in more than one factor, it was left in the factor on which it had the highest factor loading. Only when an item loaded in a different direction (e.g., had the opposite scale anchoring) in two factors was it retained in both factors. The number of items in each factor ranged from 4 to 30 with a median of 11 and 9 items in the father and mother factors, respectively. Factor loading exceeded .30 in all cases and exceeded .40 in 84% of all loadings. Between 48 and 70% of the cumulative variance was accounted for in each factor analysis.

Though the items in mother and father versions of the inventory were the same, we factor-analyzed them separately because the experience of fathers and mothers with their children is often very different, and items might therefore be grouped into different factors for the two parents. In the end, the item clusters in most factors were quite similar for mothers and fathers and the labels of factors shown in the two versions overlap for the most part. However, the item content for factors was not always the same and the differentiation is, we believe, justified. Indeed, when fathers' and mothers' data were combined and factor-analyzed together, the resultant factor groups accounted for less of the total variance than did the separate factor analysis for mothers and fathers. All statistical analyses reported were computed with factor scores assigned to individual responses.

Table 6 (Appendix B) describes the items included in each factor, the loading for each item, the mean and standard deviation of that item, and the cumulative variance accounted for by the factor. As noted in Chapter 3, three factor analyses using Kaiser Varimex rotations were done for each parent. Only factors with eigen values of 1.00 or larger were rotated. One of the analyses included items which referred predominantly to the parents' relations with each other and to their social environment outside the family. The second set of items covered the parents' behavior in relation to the child and the third set covered the child's behavior in relation to the parent. The description of items included in Table 6 (Appendix B) are somewhat abbreviated to conserve space. The scales used for most of the items are indicated in the sample from the inventory which is included as part of Chapter 3.

Table 6 describes only the factors obtained for the father's Behavior Inventory. Although there were some differences in the mother's Behavior Inventory, this table should suffice to give the reader a clear picture of the items in the inventory.

THE FAMILY COMMUNICATION TASK

This task involves parents and one child in rotating roles as senders and receivers of verbal descriptions of graphic designs like those shown in Figure 4. The task permits study of the direction and amount of information flow within the parent-child unit, as well as reflecting the accuracy with which individual members understand each other's verbal message. The game-like nature of the apparatus and situation were chosen as appealing to the largely male, 8–12 year old children in the sample.

As with other measures reported here, more than a year was spent in pilot work developing the task. Some of this pilot work is reported elsewhere by Alkire, Collum, Kaswan, and Love (1968). The task and most of the results described here were also reported by Alkire (1970). The designs were selected originally by Krauss and Glucksberg (1965) from a larger set of similar designs. The 15 designs selected by these investigators elicited a wide variety of referents from subjects who attempted to describe them. In essence, they were figures for which there are no commonly shared reference concepts. One additional design was selected for the present study using the same criterion, to make a total of 16 designs. Each design was pasted on four faces of a small 1 inch cube. The other two faces of the block were painted red and yellow. A hole was bored from the red to the yellow face so the blocks could be placed on a spindle.

The target child and his parents were seated at a table but separated from each other's view by a three-partition screen. In order to set up a communication network involving two receivers, it was necessary to use microphones and earphones so that the sender could talk privately with one receiver. The procedure allowed the sender to make an initial description of the design which both receivers could hear. The task for each receiver was to make an accurate selection of that design from the array of 16 designs he had in front of him. He could ask questions of the sender whenever he wished; however, he had to press a buzzer to signal to the sender when he wanted to make such an intervention. It was emphasized that the moment either receiver asked a question, the communication line between the sender and the other receiver was closed.

The sender was provided with a switch so that he could talk back and forth with either receiver by merely setting a lever to one of two positions. He could move the lever as often as he liked in conversing with one receiver and then the other. The setting was clearly labeled so that the sender knew which receiver he was selecting by moving the lever. The switching apparatus was connected to a masking sound (supplied by a separate tape recorder). The noise was delivered into the headset of the receiver opposite to the one which had been selected by the movement of the lever. This masking sound, started by the experimenter the moment either receiver intervened, effectively blocked any private conversation between the sender and the other receiver. No communication was possible between the two receivers at any time during the procedure.

This task was administered during the initial visit to the clinic. It included parents and target child. The child always started in the task role of sender, with his two parents serving as independent receivers. For single-parent families, of course, there was only one receiver. Each member initially had a set of three small blocks bearing practice designs which were not part of the test array of 16 designs. The three-partition screen was not yet in place so that the use of the switching apparatus could be shown. The method of description and accurate selection of the designs was explained carefully. The use of the buzzer was also demonstrated and the subjects were told of the reason for the masking sound. The introduction also emphasized the role of the sender as the initiator of the information exchange process.

All members then put on their earphones and the three-partition screen separating each family member was put into place. The staff person put the child sender's three practice blocks into his dispenser, showed him how to remove the first one, and instructed him to begin describing the design on the block to his parents. The receivers were told to make their choices by putting the chosen blocks on the spindle each had before him.

The parents were reminded to press their buzzer before talking. The masking sound was introduced when one of the parents asked a question or made a comment. If there was no parental intervention, the staff person pressed one of the buzzers, turned on the masking sound, and then demonstrated to the child the use of the lever in choosing the parent with whom he wished to speak.

At this point, the instructions were reviewed for all members. The time limit for description and selection of each design (90 seconds) was emphasized and the bell signaling the end of this trial was sounded. The child was then told to take a second practice design from the dispenser and begin describing it to his parents. On this trial, the staff person actually set the clock so that the bell would ring at he end of the 90-second limit. Corrections were made on any inappropriate task behaviors of the family members during the practice trials. Any tendency to ask questions about the design from the receiver position without pressing the buzzer was especially discouraged. The third trial run was then completed.

The practice blocks were picked up and 16 blocks representing the total array of designs were set out for each receiver. Six randomly selected designs were placed in the dispenser in front of the child. The last two of these designs were duplicates randomly selected from the first three designs. The instructions were reviewed briefly and the series of trials with the child sending was undertaken. No information was given about the accuracy of selection of the designs.

After the child's description and parents' question-answering sequence for each of the six blocks in turn had been completed, one parent (randomly selected in two-parent families) was assigned the role of sender. The child then took that parent's seat and served as an independent receiver along with the remaining parent. Following that second series of trials, the other parent took on the task role of sender while the parent who had been sending rotated to the vacated receiver's chair. In each instance after instructions were briefly reviewed, the sender transmitted six designs which had been selected following the basic procedure outlined earlier.

The number of correct choices of blocks made by each receiver for each sender was the indication of accuracy of their communication; the pattern of questioning by the receivers (either to help clarify the message or help themselves in a design choice) and the responses of the sender gave information about the communication processes within the family. The audiotapes which contain each family's verbal interchanges are still to be analyzed in detail.

VIDEOTAPING PROCEDURES

Upon arrival for their first session at the clinic, the family was shown into a large room with a standard arrangement of furniture and supplies, including toys and refreshments. They were told that this was the "family" room and were invited to make themselves comfortable until the staff member who would see them was free. After the family had been in the room for 5 minutes, a project member entered and greeted them. He asked the father (or if the family contained no father, the mother) to come with him to provide initial information (about family composition, educational levels, and similar data). Another project worker took siblings and other relatives to a different room for 10 minutes, leaving the mother and target (referred or control) child in the family room, with the video camera continuing to record their interactions. Upon the father's return, after about 3 minutes, the mother was asked out and the father and child were left in the room. Next, the target child went out with the interviewer to answer standard questions, leaving the parents together for about 3 minutes. Finally, the total family was reassembled in the family room and told by the staff member that they would begin the major procedures in a few minutes, as soon as he had completed final preparations for their session. They were reminded that the session would last about 2½ hours and would include an interview during which they would talk about the things that brought them to the clinic. They were asked whether they had discussed this problem together. Whatever their response, the staff member requested that they spend time before his return in reviewing each person's understanding of why they had come to the clinic and what each of them would like to have changed in their family. This request was given in a relatively standard (though not verbatim) text, concluding with the explanation that such a review would make the upcoming interview more productive. The staff member then excused himself to finish his preparations. Five minutes of the ensuing discussion among family members, termed the "Problem Definition," constituted the end of the videotaped interaction. The interviewer returned with three assistants whom he introduced. The parents and one consultant remained in the family room, while the target child went with a different staff member to another interview room; all three then completed their adjective ratings. The fourth staff member took the other family members to a waiting room where TV, books, and toys were provided for the duration of the session.

TEACHER ADJECTIVE RATING SCALE

Results from the 20-word scale used by teachers were analyzed in two ways. First we extracted the two factors containing the adjectives of the 10-word lists used by the other raters (Factors IB and IIB). Secondly we used two factors containing all of the 20 adjectives (Factors IA and IIA). Factor IA for the 20-word list contained the adjectives *angry, bad, bored, lazy, mean, nagging, phony, rude,* and *selfish.* Factor IIA contained the adjectives *controlling, active, calm, clear, confident, dependable, friendly, happy, patient,* and *smart.* All statistical analyses comparing R/NR, SEL, or referral categories yielded equivalent results for comparable factors from the 10- and 20-adjective lists (i.e., results IA = IB, IIA = IIB). In order to permit direct comparison of these results with the family ratings, all analyses reported here were based on the 10-adjective ratings, containing the Negative Social Impact (IB) and the Positive Social Impact (IIB) factors used with all raters.

TEACHER BEHAVIOR INVENTORY

The 142 variables of the Inventory were factor-analyzed in several ways. The analyses reported below are based on the last of four factors analyses involving responses of 111 teachers. Factor loading was sensitive to changes in the number of cases used, the number of factors rotated, and the way in which "no response" items were handled. On the whole, however, clustering of items into the 14 factors remained quite stable in these different analyses. As for the Parent Behavior Inventory, all factor loadings were above .30 and most above .40. Unfortunately, due to a clerical error, all item overlaps among the factors were not eliminated as for the Parent Behavior Inventory. Accordingly, strict independence of factors cannot be assumed and some overlap among them should be taken into account in the interpretation of results. The 14 factors accounted for 72% of the cumulative variance.

SCHOOL OBSERVATION RATINGS

Interrater agreement was assessed by an analysis of variance procedure described by Winer (1963, p. 216) in which $r_k = 1 - $ MS within/MS between. In this analysis, the within variance comes from the difference between the two judges rating each subject and the between variance contains differences among subjects in the average of the two judges' ratings. Of the total of 35 analyses (the 10 adjectives used in the three contexts and the five interaction scales), the r_k in 27 was above .70. The overall mean r_k was .77 and the range was from .29 to .96. *Phony* was the only adjective on which agreement was consistently poor. The results suggest that, for the most part, these scales have minimal ambiguity in describing overt aspects of naturally occurring behavior in the school.

In order to correct for instrument decay in the continuous use of the same instrument by a group of judges, ratings of referred and nonreferred children were always compared with the ratings given random children for an equivalent time period. Ratings of the 116 randomly chosen children in the year 1966–1967 provided a comparison group for ratings given to referred and nonreferred children during that time period; all ratings, whether initial or follow-up, were compared to the random group and standard C scores were computed with reference to this normative group. Ratings of the 40 randomly chosen children in the year 1967–1968 provided the normative group for all ratings of referred and nonreferred children during that time period. This procedure should compensate for any systematic drift in ratings over a 2 year period due to rater bias such as changes in informal hypotheses the judges may have made.

FLOW CHART OF PROCEDURES

Average time
from receipt
of referral

1. Principal asks parents whether they wish to be referred to the Psychology Clinic, notifying the clinic if they accept.

3 days
2. Parents receive a letter from the clinic briefly indicating the opportunity to participate in a program to help the child, and advising them that they will be contacted in a few days.

1 week
3. School Measures:
   a. Raters observe the child's behavior in the classroom and playground using Adjective Rating Scale.
   *b. Project member interviews teacher, requests that she fill out Adjective Rating Scale and Behavior Inventory.

1 week
4. Parents are called for initial appointment.

2 weeks
5. Initial clinic appointment:
   a. Videotaping of interactions.
      Whole family together (free interaction).
      Mother and target child.
      Father and target child.
      Problem Definition discussion (whole family).
   *b. Recall of events during Problem Definition discussion.
   *c. Family members rate behavior during Problem Definition using Adjective Rating Scale.
   *d. View videotape describing feedback intervention program.
   *e. Communication Task.
   f. Thirty-minute interview.
   g. Parents take home Behavior Inventory.

*Involves all Feedback Intervention cases and half of all other cases.

Average time
from receipt
of referral

3 weeks   †6. Home visit by two project members. Rate behavior of each family member on Adjective Rating Scale.

4 weeks   †7. Videotape ratings. Selected scenes rated separately by each parent, referred child, and two staff raters.

5–6 weeks   †8. Review of videotape and ratings. Family views whole tape and profiles of their own and staff judges' ratings, including recall ratings (often two sessions).

7 weeks   †9. Family review of school ratings by observers and teacher as well as the findings of performance on Communication Task.

8 weeks   †10. Review of Behavior Inventories with family (e.g., examine similarities and discrepancies between parents' ratings).

9 weeks   †11. School feedback. Teacher, counselor, and principal all review materials, including videotapes and all ratings.

10 weeks   †12. School conference. School personnel, parents, and consultant meet at school.

6 months   13. Follow-up: repeat 3a, 3b, 5a, 5b, 5c, 5e, 5f, and 7.

12 months   14. Follow-up: repeat procedures as in 13.

24 months   15. Follow-up: repeat procedures as in 13.

†Used only with Feedback Intervention.

Supplementary Statistics

Table 1. FRPV IQ as Related to Socioeconomic Level and Referred—Nonreferred Groups

| | Socioeconomic Level | | | | | |
| | High | | Mid | | Low | |
	R	NR	R	NR	R	NR
Father	117	114	108	111	91	98
N	11	6	24	15	5	5
Mother	110	115	101	112	90	95
N	14	6	25	15	13	7
Child	131	131	110	130	108	108
N	18	6	39	15	24	8

Table 2. Birth Order: Comparison of Social Withdrawal and Nonreferred Groups

R: Social Withdrawal:	N = 19	NR: N = 29
Only/oldest children	14 (.74)	10 (.35)
Younger children	5 (.26)	19 (.65)

Table 3. Birth Order: Comparison within Mid-Socioeconomic level only of Social Withdrawal and Nonreferred Groups

R: Social Withdrawal, Mid SEL:	N = 14	NR: N = 15
Only/oldest children	10 (.71)	5 (.33)
Younger children	4 (.29)	10 (.67)

Table 4. Family Adjective Ratings. Person Rating (Fa, Mo, Ch): Rater Effects; Referred—Nonreferred, Socioeconomic Level Analyses.[a]

	df	IB: Negative Social Impact			IIB: Positive Social Impact		
		MS	F	p<	MS	F	p<
Father is rating							
Group (R-NR)	1	33.23	11.73	.001	13.51	5.63	.05
Person rated (R)	2	15.22	13.64	.001	4.78	6.18	.01
G × R	2	1.81	1.62		4.44	5.74	.01
Error	192	1.69			1.32		
Mother is rating							
Group (R-NR)	1	23.64	7.65	.01	29.15	13.48	.05
Person rated (R)	2	9.38	6.74	.01	1.63	1.88	.05
G × R	2	1.88	.64		3.61	4.15	
Error	192	1.96			1.30		
Child is rating							
Group (R-NR)	1	25.73	9.33	.01	7.44	3.31	.10
Person rated (R)	2	5.57	5.98	.01	9.59	10.55	.001
G × R	2	0.00	0		2.07	2.28	.10
Error	192	1.95			1.36		

[a]Since there were no significant socioeconomic level results, these data are not reported.

Table 5. Family Adjective Ratings. Person Being Rated (Fa, Mo, Ch); Referred—Nonreferred, Socioeconomic Level Analyses.

		IB: Negative Social Impact			IIB: Positive Social Impact		
	df	MS	F	p<	MS	F	p<
Father is rated							
Group (R-NR)	1	22.81	14.21	.001	16.49	11.58	.001
Rater (R)	2	6.91	4.30	.05	1.18		
SEL (S)	2	0.75			4.93	3.47	.05
G × R	2	2.59			4.51	3.17	.05
G × S	2	4.30	2.68	.10	1.56		
R × S	4	1.37			0.31		
G × R × S	4	2.28			2.04		
Error	196	1.61			1.42		
Mother is rated							
Group (R-NR)	1	21.51	15.13	.001	0.04		
Rater (R)	2	3.93	2.76	.10	3.19	2.23	.20
SEL (S)	2	1.24			0.20		
G × R	2	0.16			1.04		
G × S	2	0.18			2.96		
R × S	4	2.21			1.29	2.07	.20
G × R × S	4	1.71			2.50		
Error	225	1.42			1.43		
Child is rated							
Group (R-NR)	1	33.36	15.92	.002	39.58	31.79	.001
Rater (R)	2	13.06	6.23	.01	0.18		
SEL (S)	2	3.43			3.05	2.45	.10
G × R	2	1.31			0.36		
G × S	2	0.19			1.74		
R × S	4	1.13			0.83		
G × R × S	4	2.40			1.05		
Error	230	2.10			1.25		

Table 6. Parent Behavior Inventory. Father's Responses. $N = 80$ (27 R, 24 NR, 29 Fernald School)

Relation and Factor Number	Question Number	Description*	Loading	Mean	S.D.
Fa → Mo					
I		*Hostile Disagreement*			
	88g	When want wife to do something, you get angry if she doesn't do it.	0.77	1.42	0.90
	90e	When disagree with wife, you get angry.	0.76	1.91	1.01
	90h	When disagree with wife, you keep after her to change her mind.	0.75	1.76	1.01
	88h	When want wife to do something, you say other wives do it.	0.73	1.40	0.91
	89	How often do you and wife disagree on family matters?	0.73	2.06	1.01
	90g	When disagree with wife, you let he: know you feel hurt.	0.71	1.54	0.90
	90d	When disagree with wife, you go own way without resolving issue.	0.69	1.81	1.02
	88m	When want wife to do something, you say you'll think more highly of her.	0.68	1.47	0.90
	81f	How often do you and wife argue?	0.68	2.31	1.01
	90f	When disagree with wife, you try to get around her by being nice.	0.67	1.55	0.90
	88i	When want wife to do something, you say it's for her own good.	0.66	1.74	1.06
	88f	When want wife to do something, you try to kid her into doing it.	0.58	1.84	1.12
	88b	When want wife to do something, you say you'll do something in return.	0.57	1.29	0.72
	88a	When want wife to do something, you say you would do this for her if she asked.	0.53	1.44	0.78
	88k	When want wife to do something, you say it would please you if she did it.	0.52	2.10	1.07
	88j	When want wife to do something, you ask her to do it because she is your wife.	0.51	1.61	1.02
	82	How different are your and your wife's interests and activities?	0.47	2.65	1.15
	88e	When want wife to do something, you give reasons, but leave decision to her.	0.45	2.37	1.05

Cumulative variance = .14

* Descriptions have been condensed to save space.

II Share Decision-Making and Activities

81k	How often do you and wife plan activities, make joint decisions?	0.75	3.34	0.94
81b	How often do you and wife talk about work?	0.74	3.47	0.94
81j	How often do you and wife discuss community or political events?	0.71	3.06	1.01
86	How often ask wife to do something *with you*?	0.69	3.22	0.76
81a	How often do you and wife discuss the children?	0.68	3.80	0.64
81d	How often do you and wife talk about common interests?	0.68	3.44	0.97
81c	How often do you and wife talk about social activities?	0.68	3.67	0.78
81e	How often do you and wife talk about personal matters?	0.67	3.71	0.80
85	How often do you ask wife to do something for you?	0.58	3.40	0.88
87	How often do you ask wife to do something for herself?	0.51	2.60	0.88
73c	How often do you both decide what adult friends to invite or visit?	0.49	3.05	1.18
81h	How often do you and wife watch TV?	0.49	3.94	0.65
88l	When want wife to do something, you discuss and work it out together.	0.44	2.34	1.09
88c	When want wife to do something, you give reasons, but leave decision to her.	0.41	2.38	1.05
74c	How often do you both decide how to handle children?	0.35	3.39	1.13
79b	How often does wife fix things?	0.33	2.17	1.08

Cumulative variance = .23

III Church-Home Orientation

99	How often do you go to church?	0.74	1.57	0.91
91a	How often active in church groups?	0.68	1.47	1.04
100	How often does wife go to same church?	0.65	1.74	0.96
101	How often children attend Sunday School?	0.56	2.32	1.06
78a	How often do you do gardening?	0.49	2.11	1.22
72c	How often do you and wife decide how and when money is spent in home?	0.43	3.31	1.12
79a	How often do you fix things?	0.36	2.81	1.19

Cumulative variance = .29

Table 6. (Continued)

Relation and Factor Number	Question Number	Description	Loading	Mean	S.D.
IV		*Like Neighborhood and Neighbors*			
	97	How well do people keep their homes in your neighborhood?	0.78	4.59	0.79
	96	How much do you like the neighborhood children?	0.72	3.72	0.89
	95	How much do you like the people in neighborhood?	0.70	3.65	0.89
	94	How well do you like the neighborhood in which you live?	0.65	4.07	1.16
	98	How often visit with neighborhood families?	0.41	2.32	1.16
		Cumulative variance = .35			
V		*Father's Household Activities*			
	76a	How often do you help with housework?	0.78	2.66	1.14
	77a	How often do you wash dishes?	0.73	2.36	1.19
	75a	How often do you do some cooking?	0.67	2.14	1.05
	80a	How often do you do clean-up jobs?	0.61	3.07	1.06
	79a	How often do you fix things?	0.48	2.81	1.19
		Cumulative variance = .39			
VI		*Wife's Decision Making; Husband's Activities in Community*			
	72a	How often does wife decide how and when money is spent in home?	0.58	1.77	1.06
	91f	How often are you active in organized youth groups?	0.56	1.65	0.97
	73a	How often wife decides what adult friends to invite or visit? (also F. I)	0.55	1.97	1.12
	74a	How often wife decides how to handle the children?	0.55	2.56	1.35
	72b	How often you decide when money is spent in home? (also F. VII)	0.48	2.20	1.24
	91b	How often are you active in PTA activities?	0.47	1.10	0.34
	74b	How often you decide how to handle the children? (also F. VII)	0.45	2.26	1.14
	91c	How often are you active in volunteer service activities?	0.43	1.32	0.79
		Cumulative variance = .43			

VII
Mother's Household Activities

75b	How often does wife do some cooking?	0.80	4.59	0.74
76b	How often does wife help with housework?	0.80	4.46	0.91
77b	How often does wife wash dishes?	0.80	4.27	1.10
73b	How often you decide what adult friends to invite or visit?	−0.40	1.70	0.80
74b	How often you decide to handle children?	−0.41	2.26	1.14
72b	How often you decide how and when money is spent in home?	−0.44	2.20	1.24
	Cumulative variance = .47			

VIII
Wife Decides Disagreements—Joint Decisions

90b	When disagree with wife, you give in after presenting your point of view.	0.66	2.06	0.88
90a	When disagree with wife, you give in without discussion.	0.63	1.71	0.80
73c	How often you and wife decide what adult friends to invite or visit?	0.57	3.05	1.18
81m	How often do you and wife have adult company in?	0.57	2.16	0.68
811	How often do you and wife go out together?	0.52	2.75	0.72
72c	How often you and wife decide how and when money is spent in home?	0.36	3.31	1.12
	Cumulative variance = .50			

IX
Child's Household Activities

77c	How often does child wash dishes?	−0.75	2.34	1.19
76c	How often does child help with housework?	−0.68	3.04	1.04
80c	How often does child do clean-up jobs?	−0.65	3.12	1.01
79c	How often does child fix things?	−0.47	1.54	0.86
75c	How often does child do some cooking?	−0.39	2.00	0.98
	Cumulative variance = .53			

Fa → Ch
I
Affectionate Behavior

33d	How often do you show affection to child when he is helpful to you?	0.86	3.35	0.97
33b	How often do you show affection to child when he does more than expected?	0.81	3.34	1.01

Table 6. (Continued)

Relation and Factor Number	Question Number	Description	Loading	Mean	S.D.
	34b	How often do you tell your child you like him?	0.79	3.67	0.88
	33a	How often do you show affection to child when he does what is expected?	0.78	3.50	0.86
	33h	How often do you show affection to child for no special reason?	0.75	3.51	1.01
	33c	How often do you show affection to child when gets a good grade?	0.73	3.10	1.32
	33j	How often do you show affection to child when he is sick or hurts self?	0.72	3.19	1.39
	33f	How often do you show affection to child when he does not misbehave?	0.69	2.92	1.21
	33e	How often do you show affection to child when you are blue or unhappy?	0.68	2.26	1.17
	33i	How often do you show affection to child when you think he needs it?	0.65	3.29	1.15
	34a	How often do you hug or kiss your child?	0.62	3.47	1.15
	22h	How often does child talk to you about something he wants from you?	0.53	3.24	0.82
	33g	How often do you show affection to child when you want him to do something for you?	0.52	2.42	1.20
	34c	How often do you do something with your child or for him?	0.47	3.17	0.82
	40b	When you want your child to do something, how often do you tell him he should do as you ask because you know what is best?	0.46	3.00	0.98
	34g	How often do you joke with your child?	0.39	3.56	0.81
	34e	How often do you let your child do what he wants?	0.34	2.92	0.90
	61c	When child does something wrong, how often do you explain what he was doing wrong?	0.34	3.10	0.96

Cumulative variance = .16

Ignore, Physically Isolate Child

63a	When child has done something wrong, how often does he stay in his room for less than an hour?	0.60	1.92	0.90
63b	When child has done something wrong, how often does he stay in his room for several hours?	0.58	1.45	0.76
60a	When child has done something wrong, how often do you take away privileges for a day or less?	0.54	1.85	0.76
57c	When you are angry with child, how often do you show your anger by going to your room?	0.52	1.37	0.82
62a	When child does something wrong, how often do you ignore him for less than an hour?	0.48	1.35	0.71
66d	When you see child do something wrong, how often do you wait for spouse to come home?	0.41	1.17	0.55
19	Time spent with child at home evenings?	−0.50	3.00	0.84
20	How many nights spent at home during week?	−0.60	3.39	0.77

Cumulative variance = .26

III

Understand Child, See Child as Similar to Wife

36b	How much do you think child is like your wife as a person in intelligence?	−0.67	3.24	1.12
36c	How much do you think child is like your wife as a person in expression of feelings?	−0.60	3.46	1.18
36a	How much do you think child is like your wife as a person in looks?	−0.37	2.76	1.19
37	How often are you fairly concerned what child's feelings really are?	−0.36	3.61	0.89
38	How often are you fairly sure what your child really means by things he says?	−0.36	3.91	0.77
66a	When you see your child do something wrong, how often do you punish him immediately?	0.40	2.64	1.17

Cumulative variance = .31

Table 6. (Continued)

Relation and Factor Number	Question Number	Description	Loading	Mean	S.D.
IV		*Child's Communication*			
	22b	How often does child talk to you about what went on during day?	0.77	3.46	0.89
	22a	How often does child talk to you about school work?	0.73	3.11	1.07
	22c	How often does child talk to you about other people?	0.63	3.26	0.82
	22d	How often does child talk to you about problems he has?	0.60	2.80	1.08
	34f	How often do you tussle or fight with your child?	0.56	2.80	1.01
	18d	How often do you wrestle or roughhouse with your child?	0.49	2.61	0.97
	22g	How often does child talk to you about something good that happened?	0.46	3.46	0.69
	18g	How often do you read to your child?	0.41	1.87	1.04
	35c	How much is your child like you as a person in expression of feelings?	0.39	3.41	1.21
	18h	How often do you help your child with his homework?	0.38	2.74	1.08
	22e	How often does child talk to you about a lot of different things?	0.35	3.66	0.78
	84	How different are you and another child's activities and interests?	−0.48	2.54	0.98
		Cumulative variance = .35			
V		*Personalized, Referent Influence Attempts*			
	40h	When want child to do something, how often do you tell him you would be hurt if he didn't do it?	0.71	1.95	1.03
	40m	When want child to do something, how often do you let him know that at his age you would have done what you are asking him to do?	0.68	1.99	1.12
	40l	When want child to do something, how often do you let him know that you would yourself do what you are asking?	0.67	2.51	1.14
	40i	When want child to do something, how often do you tell him if he does what you ask, you will do something for him?	0.67	1.77	0.95
	40g	When want child to do something, how often do you tell him you would think more highly of him?	0.65	2.60	1.11

40n	When want child to do something, how often do you tell him it is your duty to ask him to do this?	0.60	2.00	1.14
40f	When want child to do something, how often do you tell him that it would please you?	0.56	2.94	0.96
40o	When want child to do something, how often do you let him know that if he doesn't do it, you will have to tell his mother?	0.50	1.19	0.55
40c	When want child to do something, how often do you tell him what you are asking is no different than what other children have to do?	0.47	2.47	1.07
40d	When you want child to do something, how often do you tell him that he will be punished if he doesn't do it?	0.43	2.75	1.04
40k	When you want child to do something, how often do you try to kid him into doing what you ask?	0.39	2.05	1.03
70a	How often do you leave the children alone when child quarrels with his siblings?	−0.34	2.56	1.15

Cumulative variance = .38

Know Child

VI				
39a	To what extent do you know what child is doing when playing outside the home?	−0.71	3.56	1.00
39c	To what extent do you know with whom he plays and what he does when you're not there?	−0.61	3.84	0.89
39b	To what extent do you know things your child is doing in school?	−0.58	3.45	0.93
23	How often do you do things with child that he enjoys?	−0.57	2.92	0.90
21	Time spent in activity with child on weekends?	−0.56	3.26	0.96
18i	How often do you teach your child new things?	−0.49	2.64	0.97
18a	How often do you go camping with your child?	−0.46	1.62	0.62
19	Time spent with child at home evenings?	−0.41	3.00	0.84
24	How often do you do things with child you enjoy?	−0.40	2.89	0.90
18c	How often do you play ball with your child?	−0.40	2.36	1.03
34g	How often do you joke with child?	−0.39	3.56	0.81
34d	How often do you give your child presents?	−0.35	1.80	0.77
59	How often do you carry through with punishment?	−0.34	3.84	0.77
83	How different are you and child's activities and interests?	0.50	2.49	1.06

Cumulative variance = .42

Table 6. (Continued)

Relation and Factor Number	Question Number	Description	Loading	Mean	S.D.
VII		*Punish Aggressive Behavior*			
	68c	When your child quarrels with other children, how often do you step in if fighting gets rough?	0.75	1.92	1.18
	68b	When your child quarrels with other children, how often do step in before a real fight begins?	0.75	1.97	1.11
	68d	When your child quarrels with other children, how often do you punish child for fighting?	0.71	1.39	0.72
	70b	When child quarrels with sibs, how often do you step in before a real fight starts?	0.55	2.95	1.11
	66b	When see child doing wrong, how often make sure he knows what he did wrong, then punish?	0.47	2.94	1.13
	70d	When child quarrels with sibs, how often do you punish child for fighting?	0.45	2.01	0.97
	70c	When child quarrels with sibs, how often do you step in only if fighting gets violent?	0.42	2.37	1.33
	66a	When see child doing wrong, how often punish immediately?	0.39	2.64	1.17
	61b	When child does something wrong, how often do you spank him so he really feels it?	0.38	1.67	0.85
	66c	When see child doing something wrong, how often wait until not angry, then punish?	0.36	1.95	1.07
		Cumulative variance = .45			
VIII		*Parental Anger*			
	57h	When angry with child, show anger by shaming him?	0.65	1.62	0.79
	61e	When child has done something wrong, how often yell at him?	0.65	2.42	0.99
	57b	When angry with child, show anger by yelling?	0.63	2.52	1.06
	57a	When angry with child, tell him off?	0.56	2.52	0.98

58	How often threaten to punish child?	0.56	2.29	0.84
57i	When angry with child, ignore him?	0.53	1.40	0.82
57g	When angry with child, strike or hit him?	0.49	1.64	0.73
61f	When child done something wrong, make him feel ashamed?	0.46	1.76	0.86
61d	When child has done something wrong, scold him?	0.46	2.99	0.86
61a	When child has done something wrong, give him light slap?	0.45	1.75	0.92
61b	When child has done something wrong, how often spank so he really feels it?	0.35	1.67	0.85
64	To what extent does your punishment make child behave better?	−0.35	3.42	1.29

Cumulative variance = .48

Ch → Fa
I

Avoids Personal Confrontations

30f	If refuse to do what child asks, he gets sullen?	−0.76	2.06	1.15
30h	If refuse to do what child asks, he acts hurt and leaves?	−0.69	2.10	1.09
28f	How often does child ask—tell you parents of friends do this?	−0.68	1.76	0.98
31d	How often does child go to his room?	−0.66	2.09	1.01
31a	How often does child sulk?	−0.65	2.04	1.07
16e	How often does child show fear?	−0.62	1.87	1.00
30c	If refuse to do what child asks, he cries, complains? (also F. III)	−0.60	2.02	1.06
30g	If refuse to do what child asks, he goes to wife?	−0.57	2.30	1.15
28h	How often does child ask—says he has the right to do this?	−0.54	1.59	0.98
29	How often do you refuse child something?	−0.53	2.59	1.03
28e	How often does child ask—promises to be good?	−0.52	2.07	1.09
43e	When ask child to do something other than regular chores, to what extent will he do it if promise to give him something? (also F. XIV)	−0.50	1.86	1.29
16h	How often does child say people don't like him?	−0.50	1.80	0.96
56d	How often child spends extra money by buying presents for family?	−0.47	1.42	0.81
55b	When child wants money outside of allowance, he asks father?	−0.46	2.06	1.08
55a	When child wants money outside of allowance, he asks mother?	−0.46	2.12	1.08
17b	How often does child talk back to adults outside family?	−0.46	1.52	1.02

Table 6. (Continued)

Relation and Factor Number	Question Number	Description	Loading	Mean	S.D.
	13h	How often does child get tense and worried?	−0.45	2.50	1.18
	32c	How often does child show affection when he wants you to do something? (also F. II)	−0.40	2.52	1.19
	16a	How often does child bite his nails?	−0.40	1.57	1.19
	28b	How often does child ask—suggests indirectly?	−0.38	2.04	1.04
	16i	How often does child act ashamed for something he has done?	−0.37	1.76	0.83
		Cumulative variance = .13			
II		*Affectionate Behavior*			
	32f	How often does child show affection for no special reason?	−0.78	2.89	1.15
	31i	How often does child hug or kiss you?	−0.77	3.12	1.23
	32a	How often does child show affection when he is happy?	−0.75	3.51	0.98
	31j	How often does child tell you he likes you?	−0.74	2.94	1.04
	32b	How often does child show affection when he has gotten what he wanted?	−0.66	3.14	1.13
	31m	How often does child tussle with you?	−0.63	3.00	1.02
	31l	How often does child tease and joke with you?	−0.57	3.25	0.96
	31k	How often does child do something he knows you will like?	−0.51	2.82	0.90
	32d	How often does child show affection when he feels badly?	−0.46	2.20	1.07
	32e	How often does child show affection when he wants attention?	−0.43	2.56	1.13
	32c	How often does child show affection when wants you to do something? (also F. I)	−0.39	2.52	1.19
		Cumulative variance = .21			

III   *Hostile, Defiant Behavior*

Item	Question			
31c	How often does child yell?	−0.82	2.02	1.20
17a	How often does child talk back to adults in family?	−0.69	2.69	1.32
30e	If refuse to do what child ask, he gets angry?	−0.68	2.12	1.14
28c	How often does child ask—demands?	−0.67	1.59	1.09
45e	How often does child complain about rules, chores—threatens to refuse to follow?	−0.59	1.74	1.03
15k	How often does child have temper tantrums?	−0.59	2.00	1.09
30b	If refuse to do what child asks, he keeps after you, nags?	−0.58	2.52	1.20
45b	How often does child complain about rules, chores—argues?	−0.58	2.50	1.19
69	To what extent child fights with sibs?	−0.58	3.30	1.12
14g	How much does child react when doesn't get his own way?	−0.57	3.74	1.02
31b	How often does child tell you off?	−0.57	1.54	0.86
14i	How much does he react when he is corrected or criticized?	−0.55	3.51	1.07
45d	How often does child complain about rules, chores—refuses to follow rule? (also F. XIV)	−0.55	1.82	1.06
30c	If you refuse to do what child asks, he cries, complains? (also F. I)	−0.49	2.02	1.06
31h	How often does child strike or hit?	−0.44	1.34	0.83
45f	How often does child complain about rules, chores—ignores, does what he wants? (also F. VIII)	−0.43	1.74	0.85
31g	How often does child cry? (also F. XII)	−0.42	2.10	1.09
31f	How often does child throw or break things?	−0.41	1.21	0.52
28a	How often does child ask—asks you directly?	−0.39	3.15	1.06
15h	How often does child do his work poorly?	−0.37	2.95	1.07
30a	If you refuse to do what child asks, he accepts your first answer?	+0.44	2.76	1.03
43a	When ask child to do something other than regular chores, to what extent will he do it immediately?	+0.44	2.95	1.07

Cumulative variance = .25

Table 6. (Continued)

Factor Number	Question Number	Description	Loading	Mean	S.D.
IV		*Economic Initiative, Social Adaptiveness*			
	55d	When child wants money outside of allowance, he gets it doing jobs for others?	−0.72	1.50	0.80
	26a	How often child does jobs to earn money?	−0.63	2.42	1.13
	50	How often does your child offer to help relatives or neighbors?	−0.60	1.90	0.95
	55e	When child wants money outside allowance, he gets it by selling things that belong to him?	−0.59	1.29	0.60
	56a	How often child spends extra money for buying toys, models?	−0.54	2.07	0.88
	56c	How often child spends extra money for buying treats for other children?	−0.50	2.01	0.88
	55c	When child wants money outside allowance, he gets it by doing extra jobs for parents?	−0.49	1.90	0.39
	9c	How often does child play with other children?	−0.42	4.29	0.64
	10a	How much does child follow others 1-5 lead group?	−0.40	3.20	1.32
	10b	How much does child find it hard to make friends 1-5 makes friends easily?	−0.37	3.86	1.11
	26b	How often child does jobs because he wants something from you?	−0.36	1.85	0.87
	56e	How often child spends extra money for—spends it, but don't know for what?	−0.34	1.50	0.75
		Cumulative variance = .29			
V		*Sensitive to Ridicule, Somatic Complaints*			
	14a	How much does child react when laughed at by adults?	−0.74	3.92	1.22
	14b	How much does child react when laughed at by children?	−0.73	4.05	1.17
	151	How often does child complain something hurts him?	−0.57	2.16	1.07
	16g	How often does child not feel well?	−0.57	1.69	0.87
	15b	How often does child whine and complain? (also F. XII)	−0.47	3.01	1.13

Item	Description			
15d	How often does child get fidgety?	−0.46	3.19	1.20
16c	How often does child sleep poorly?	−0.42	1.36	0.66
14e	How much does child react when interrupted?	−0.41	3.51	1.06
14j	How much does he react when feels promises not kept?	−0.39	4.04	0.83
14m	How much does he react when alone?	−0.38	2.45	1.26
15i	How often does child go to mother for comfort?	−0.38	2.77	0.95
14f	How much does child react when feels someone is unfair?	−0.36	4.34	0.84
8	Time at uninteresting work? minute 1-5 long as necessary.	+0.52	1.87	0.89
	Cumulative variance = .33			

VI Task Oriented, Independent

Item	Description			
44	How well does a job get done? sloppily 1-5 carefully.	0.75	3.51	0.90
12h	How much does child react when doing things by himself? doesn't 1-5 extremely happy.	0.69	3.34	1.07
27	How well does child do a job? sloppily 1-5 carefully.	0.68	3.57	1.04
51	When child does job for relatives, etc., how well does it get done? sloppily 1-5 carefully.	0.61	3.40	1.25
7	Time at interesting work? a minute 1-5 as long as necessary.	0.57	3.85	1.06
12k	How much does child react when building things? doesn't 1-5 extremely happy.	0.55	3.86	1.02
5	How good is child with his hands? poor 1-5 good.	0.50	3.75	1.20
14h	How much does child react when doesn't do well? doesn't 1-5 extremely upset.	0.48	3.74	1.03
12i	How much does child react when helps others? doesn't 1-5 extremely happy.	0.47	3.79	1.06
12d	How much does child react when given responsibility? doesn't 1-5 extremely happy.	0.46	3.60	1.05
43b	When ask child to do something other than regular chores, to what extent will he do it later (without further urging)?	0.45	2.40	1.06
12g	How much does child react when takes trips?	0.40	4.35	0.83
49	How often do relatives, etc., ask child to do something for them?	0.38	1.75	0.80
	Cumulative variance = .37			

Table 6. (Continued)

Factor Number	Question Number	Description	Loading	Mean	S.D.
VII		*Enthusiastic — Responsible*			
	13c	How often does child show enthusiasm?	0.80	4.15	0.94
	13e	How often does child clown, play around?	0.76	4.27	0.87
	13a	How often does chil `l laugh?	0.72	4.25	0.80
	13d	How often does child get excited?	0.72	3.91	1.13
	13b	How often does child whistle, sing or dance?	0.52	3.65	1.03
	13f	How often does child do chores without being reminded?	0.48	2.91	0.98
	28g	How often does child ask—shows good objective reasons why?	0.35	2.21	0.91
	13g	How often does child do homework without being reminded?	0.32	2.94	0.96
		Cumulative variance = .40			
VIII		*Interpersonal Responsiveness*			
	14c	How much does child react when scolded? upset?	−0.61	3.96	1.11
	14d	How much does child react when spanked? upset?	−0.57	4.14	1.18
	12b	How much does child react when gets presents?	−0.53	4.44	0.73
	12f	How much does child react when father spends time with him?	−0.52	4.21	0.84
	11	How often is child happy?	−0.51	3.99	0.75
	14k	How much does child react when nobody pays attention to him? upset?	−0.51	3.46	1.15
	12c	How much does child react when gets affection?	−0.37	4.12	0.92
	9d	How often does child play with pets?	0.36	3.64	1.29
	45f	How often child complains about rules, chores—ignores rule, does what he wants? (also F. III)	0.44	1.74	0.85
		Cumulative variance = .43			

IX. Autonomy and Independence

71a	How often does child decide what he should wear?	0.70	3.62	0.92
71c	How often does child decide who he can have as friends?	0.69	3.59	1.14
71d	How often does child decide when and where he can play?	0.63	3.45	0.98
71b	How often does child decide when he should do his homework?	0.52	2.99	1.24
9b	How often does child decide when he should play with sibs?	0.39	4.04	1.04

Cumulative variance = .46

X. Displaced Aggression

12n	How much does child react when taking things apart? (happy)	−0.63	3.01	1.15
56b	How often does child spend extra money on food and candy?	−0.49	2.69	1.09
12m	How much does child react when breaking things? (happy)	−0.45	2.12	0.93
12e	How much does child react when mother spends time with him? (happy)	0.36	3.94	0.96

Cumulative variance = .48

XI. Interpersonal Activity Level

4	How good is child at athletics?	−0.58	3.54	1.22
1	How active is child?	−0.52	4.22	0.97
2	How much does child talk?	−0.44	3.95	0.94
3	How noisy is child? (also F. XV)	−0.44	3.22	1.12
5a	How often does child play alone?	0.61	2.09	1.26
45c	How often does child complain to mother about rules and chores?	0.34	2.07	1.16

Cumulative variance = .51

XII. Cries, Whines

15n	How often does child try to get someone else in trouble?	−0.56	2.14	1.06
15b	How often does he whine and complain? (also F. V)	−0.53	3.01	1.13
15c	How often does he get angry?	−0.47	3.16	1.12
15m	How often does child blame someone else for difficulty?	−0.47	2.84	0.89
15a	How often does child cry?	−0.43	2.51	1.02
15f	How often does child get extra quiet? (also F. XIII)	−0.43	2.12	0.96

269

Table 6. (Continued)

Factor Number	Question Number	Description	Loading	Mean	S.D.
XII					
	31g	How often does child act toward you in the following ways: cries? (also F. III)	−0.41	2.10	1.09
	17c	How often does child take things that don't belong to him?	−0.35	1.56	0.93
	12a	How much does child react when praised?	−0.33	4.21	0.92
	71e	How often does child decide when and what he should watch on TV?	0.37	3.46	0.95
	71f	How often does child decide when he should go to bed?	0.46	2.04	1.11
	14l	How much does child react when someone else gets hurt?	0.61	3.60	1.12
		Cumulative variance = .53			
XIII		*Solitary Play*			
	16j	How often does child daydream?	−0.67	2.27	1.16
	26d	How often does child do jobs because he is bored?	−0.54	1.69	0.87
	15g	How often does child get silly?	−0.52	3.25	1.07
	28d	How often does child ask you for something by being especially affectionate?	−0.50	2.29	1.16
	25	How often does child say he wants to help you?	−0.44	2.64	0.98
	15e	How often does child go off by himself?	−0.41	2.41	1.08
	15f	How often does child get extra quiet? (also F. XII)	−0.41	2.12	0.96
	16k	How often does child play with imaginary characters?	−0.41	1.70	1.12
	26c	How often does child do jobs because he feels guilty and wants to make up?	−0.41	1.65	0.87
	26e	How often does child do jobs for no special reason?	−0.39	2.11	1.01
	17i	How many different children does child play with?	0.39	2.94	0.46
		Cumulative variance = .55			

XIV. Inconsistent Discipline of Child

47	How often do you change the rules?	0.63	1.97	0.89
43d	When you ask child to do something other than regular chores, to what extent will he do it only if you threaten him?	0.55	2.46	1.39
43c	When you ask child to do something other than regular chores, to what extent will he do it after you urge him?	0.54	2.96	1.08
45d	How often does child complain about rules and chores by refusing to comply? (also F. III)	0.42	1.82	1.06
46	How often does child have good reason to object to your rules?	0.41	1.75	0.79
43e	When you ask child to do something other than regular chores, to what extent will he do it if you promise to give him something? (F. I)	0.41	1.86	1.29
48	How often does child have a right to be angry with you?	0.41	1.77	0.83
41c	How often does child follow rules and do chores after being threatened?	0.40	2.82	1.28
45a	How often does child complain about rules and chores by talking with you about objections?	0.36	2.51	0.98
41b	How often does child follow rules and chores after being reminded?	0.34	3.62	0.83
12j	How much does child react when he hurts others? (happy)	-0.33	1.89	0.84
	Cumulative variance = .57			

XV. Verbal Hostility

17h	How often does child threaten to hurt other children?	-0.64	1.35	0.68
3	How noisy is child? (also F. XI)	-0.62	3.22	1.12
31e	How often does child act toward you in the following ways: leaves the house?	-0.43	1.31	0.67
67	To what extent does child quarrel with other children?	-0.40	2.01	0.95
	Cumulative variance = .59			

Table 7. Videotape Analysis—Study 1: Comparison of Referred and Control Samples

		R	NR	Difference
Child IQ[a]	Mean	120	125	$t = 1.02$
	S.D.	(12)	(12)	
Child age	Mean	9.85	8.90	$t = 1.79(*)$
Child sex	% male	85%	70%	$X^{2b} = 1.02$
Family Composition	% two-parent	45%	00%	$X^{2b} = 4.46*$
Occupation of household head[c]	Mean	4.11	4.22	$t = 0.17$
	S.D.	(1.51)	(1.48)	
Education of household head[c]	Mean	3.41	3.40	$t = 0.02$
	S.D.	(1.15)	(1.11)	

[a]Measured by Ammons Full-Range Vocabulary Test; this instrument was used in order to reduce academic and cultural weightings even though it gives inflated IQ values.

[b]Adjusted by Yates' correction for small samples.

[c]Hollingshead (Hollingshead & Redlich, 1958) seven-point scales (1 = high status; 7 = low status) for occupational and educational status.

(*) $p < .10$.

*$p < .05$.

Table 8. Videotape Analysis—Study 1: Inter-Correlation between Dimensions (First 5 Minutes)

	Directing	Positive Evaluation	Evaluative Range
Activity			
Referred mother ($n = 18$)	+.36	+.19	+.27
Nonreferred mother ($n = 10$)	+.46	+.47	−.08
Referred father ($n = 13$)	+.04	+.81**	+.41
Nonreferred father ($n = 10$)	−.06	+.27	−.43
Referred child ($n = 20$)	+.46	+.51	−.06
Nonreferred child ($n = 10$)	+.38	+.52	+.34
Directing			
Referred mother	—	−.41	+.10
Nonreferred mother	—	−.11	+.13
Referred father	—	−.07	+.42
Nonreferred father	—	+.34	+.34
Referred child	—	+.02	+.34
Nonreferred child	—	+.49	+.07

Table 8. (Continued)

	Directing	Positive Evaluation	Evaluative Range
Positive evaluation			
Referred mother	—	—	−.19
Nonreferred mother	—	—	−.50
Referred father	—	—	+.47
Nonreferred father	—	—	+.51
Referred child	—	—	−.66**
Nonreferred child	—	—	+.22

$**p < .01.$

Table 9. Correlation of Talkativeness with Other Dimensions (First 5 Minutes)

	Activity	Directing	Positive Evaluation	Evaluative Range
Mother				
Referred ($n = 18$)	+.65**	+.26	+.05	+.44
Nonreferred ($n = 10$)	+.56	+.01	+.48	−.57
Father				
Referred ($n = 13$)	+.47	−.19	+.41	+.51
Nonreferred ($n = 10$)	+.23	+.58	+.49	+.13
Child				
Referred ($n = 20$)	+.02	+.08	−.09	+.10
Nonreferred ($n = 10$)	+.30	+.75**	+.33	+.21

$**p = .01.$

Table 10. Differences between Referred and Nonreferred Families

	Referred		Nonreferred		
	M	σ	M	σ	Difference
Mother					
Activity	1.91	0.78	2.05	0.55	−0.14
Directing	1.47	0.78	1.38	0.90	+0.09
Evaluation	+0.27	0.85	+0.66	0.43	−0.39
Evaluative Range	2.60	1.38	2.20	0.78	+0.40
Talking[a]	66	38	76	32	−0.10
Father					
Activity	1.74	0.61	1.54	0.56	+0.20
Directing	1.19	0.51	0.64	0.60	+0.55*
Evaluation	+0.60	0.89	+0.42	0.43	+0.18
Evaluative Range	2.44	0.85	1.20	0.54	+1.24**
Talking	53	28	29	18	+0.24*

273

Table 10. (Continued)

	Referred		Nonreferred		
	M	σ	M	σ	Difference
Child					
Activity	3.17	1.02	3.07	0.85	+0.10
Directing	0.77	0.51	0.59	0.74	+0.18
Evaluation	+0.35	0.89	+0.38	0.26	−0.03
Evaluative range	2.21	1.16	1.15	0.36	+1.06**
Talking	41	29	27	20	+0.14

[a]Seconds talked during 5 minutes
*p < .05.
**p < .01.

Note: Comparisons were made within the referred sample of one-parent versus two-parent families as a possible artifact in observed differences: no significant differences (or trends) were found on any of the dimensions measured.

Table 11. Intercorrelations between Ratings of Child Behavior and Ratings of Parental Behavior (First 5 Minutes)

	Father-Child (n = 23)	Mother-Child (n = 28)
Activity	−.03	−.38*
Directing	+.45*	−.10
Evaluation	−.02	+.02
Talking	+.41*	+.18
Evaluative range	+.78**	+.20

*p < .05.
**p < .01.

Table 12. Relationships between Behavior of Family Members[a] and Referral Problem of Child

	Severity Rating On:			
	Aggressiveness	Hyperactivity	Social Withdrawal	Poor Attention Control
Mother (n = 18)				
Activity	−.05	−.25	−.04	−.10
Directing	−.12	+.30	+.23	+.07
Evaluation	.00	−.20	+.06	−.22
Talking	+.04	−.06	+.27	+.18
Evaluative Range	+.01	−.37	−.11	−.01

Table 12. (Continued)

	Severity Rating On:			
	Aggressiveness	Hyperactivity	Social Withdrawal	Poor Attention Control
Father ($n = 13$)				
Activity	−.44	+.28	+.06	+.19
Directing	+.38	+.09	−.26	+.29
Evaluation	−.65*	+.33	+.04	+.07
Talking	−.15	+.34	+.81**	+.49
Evaluative Range	+.09	+.34	+.13	+.60*
Child ($n = 20$)				
Activity	−.16	+.33	+.08	+.53*
Directing	−.36	+.08	−.08	+.03
Evaluation	+.29	+.20	−.07	+.49*
Talking	−.25	−.10	+.43	+.07
Evaluative Range	−.43	+.16	+.26	−.08

^aDuring first 5 minutes of interaction.
*$p < .05$.
**$p < .01$.

Table 13. Videotapes—Study 2: Reliability of Judges

Interjudge agreement on channel ratings of evaluative content was estimated by

$$1 - \frac{\text{mean sum of squares within scenes}}{\text{mean sum of squares between scenes}}$$

(Winer, 1962, p. 178). This formula is equivalent to the Spearman-Brown prophery formula. Reliability coefficients (based on a range of 67 independent messages) were +.93 for verbal content, +.81 for vocal content, and +.93 for visual content.

Table 14. Proportion of Referred and Nonreferred Families Producing Conflicting Messages

		Conflict^a	No Conflict	Total
Disturbed	n	12	8	20
	Proportion	(.67)	(.33)	
Normal	n	3	7	10
	Proportion	(.30)	(.70)	
Total	n	15	15	30

^aA family was categorized as "conflicting" if either parent produced at least one conflicting message (there were potentially four messages per family, two for each parent); a family was categorized as "non-conflicting" if neither message by either parent contained channel conflict. The unit of analysis was the family, not the message.

Table 15. Proportion of Conflicting Messages Produced by Mothers and Fathers (Referred versus Nonreferred Groups)

		Conflict[a]	No Conflict	Total[b]
Mothers				
Referred	n	10	7	17
	Proportion	(.59)	(.42)	
Nonreferred	n	1	9	10
	Proportion	(.10)	(.90)	
Total	n	11	16	27
Fathers				
Referred	n	2	10	12
	Proportion	(.17)	(.83)	
Nonreferred	n	3	6	9
	Proportion	(.33)	(.67)	
Total	n	5	16	21

[a] A parent was categorized as "conflicting" if he produced at least one conflicting message; a parent was categorized as "nonconflicting" if neither of his messages contained channel conflict. The unit of analysis was the individual parent.

[b] The f's do not add to the total N (30 sets of parents) because (a) nine families contained only one parent (b) three parents produced no agreed-upon evaluative messages.

Table 16. Teacher Adjective Ratings: Means

	IB: Negative Social Impact			IIB: Positive Social Impact			
	Average Child	Target Child	How Child Will Rate	Average Child	Target Child	How Child Will Rate	N
Socioeconomic Level							
Hi							
Referred	4.51	5.08	4.61	4.65	3.54	5.05	15
Nonreferred	4.26	2.27	3.54	4.76	5.89	5.92	5
Mid							
Referred	4.79	4.90	4.41	4.45	3.28	4.73	31
Nonreferred	4.69	3.21	4.05	4.38	5.27	4.35	15
Lo							
Referred	4.57	6.13	5.10	4.42	4.08	4.98	17
Nonreferred	4.00	3.61	4.23	5.18	4.73	5.74	7
Referral Category							
Aggression	4.39	6.14	4.71	4.84	4.03	4.99	13
Hyperactive	4.21	6.28	4.91	4.76	3.55	4.79	11
Social Withdrawal	4.84	4.06	4.39	4.55	3.36	4.80	12
Attention Control	4.90	4.99	4.66	4.21	3.43	4.89	27

Table 17. Teacher Adjective Ratings. R, NR × SEL Analyses of Variance

		IB: Negative Social Impact			IIB: Positive Social Impact		
	df	MS	F	p	MS	F	p
Average child							
Group (R, NR)	1	1.49	ns		1.11	ns	
SEL	2	1.63	ns		1.14	ns	
G × SEL	2	0.36	ns		1.17	ns	
Error	83	1.14			0.70		
Target child							
Group (R, NR)	1	86.97	34.19	.01	43.82	26.06	.01
SEL	2	6.97	2.74	.05	1.05	0.62	
G × SEL	2	2.28	0.89		3.96	2.35	
Error	84	2.54	1.68				
How child will rate							
Group (R, NR)	1	9.45	6.30	.05	8.87	9.52	.001
SEL	2	1.71	ns		1.38		
G × SEL	2	0.87	ns		0.10		
Error	84	1.50	ns		0.93		

Table 18. Teacher Adjective Ratings. Referral Category

		IB: Negative Social Impact			
	df	MS	F	p<	IIB: Positive Social Impact
Groups	3	13.56	5.34	.01	Nonsignificant
Error	59	2.54			

Table 19A. Child's Adjective Ratings of Teacher: Means

	Hi SEL		Mid SEL		Lo SEL	
	R	NR	R	NR	R	NR
IB: negative social impact	5.47	5.48	4.40	6.12	4.95	5.97
IIB: positive social impact	5.51	6.04	5.16	6.06	5.46	6.30
IB − mid R − NR = t = 3.36						

Table 19B. Child's Adjective Ratings of Teacher: Analysis of Variance

		IB: Negative Social Impact			IIB: Positive Social Impact		
	df	MS	F	p<	MS	F	p<
Group (R − NR)	1	5.45	2.17	.20	9.22	3.67	.10
SEL	2	0.80			0.51		
G × S	2	1.17			0.19		
Error	74	2.51			2.51		

Table 20. Teacher Behavior Inventory

Factor Number	Question Number	Description	Loading	Mean	S.D.
I		*Interpersonal Conflict*			
	22g	How often do other children attack him verbally?	−0.80	2.26	1.21
	32e	If you refuse to do what he asks: he demands.	−0.75	1.98	1.13
	32d	If you refuse to do what he asks: he gets angry.	−0.71	2.13	1.24
	22f	How often do other children attack him physically?	−0.70	1.84	1.13
	22h	How often do other children threaten or bully him?	−0.70	1.79	1.04
	32b	If you refuse to do what he asks: he keeps after you, nags.	−0.67	2.36	1.35
	18	How often does child get angry?	−0.65	2.67	1.27
	19a	How often does child show anger by sulking?	−0.64	2.81	1.36
	17c	How often does child show worry by getting angry?	−0.64	2.88	1.31
	32f	If you refuse to do what he asks: he gets sullen.	−0.63	2.41	1.34
	22b	How often do other children tease or "pick" on him?	−0.63	2.01	1.15
	24g	How does child attempt to win acceptance from teacher: telling on others?	−0.61	2.59	1.31
	23d	How does child attempt to win acceptance from peers: bullying, threatening?	−0.60	2.21	1.42
	19e	How often does child show anger: attacks other? (also in X)	−0.59	2.08	1.37
	19b	How often does child show anger: tells you off?	−0.57	1.59	1.05
	28c	Under what conditions does he come to you: when he has a complaint? (also in III)	−0.57	3.28	1.23
	21f	How often does child threaten or hurt other children?	−0.56	2.01	1.40
	16e	How upset does child get when interrupted in some activity?	−0.51	2.80	1.14
	23h	How does child attempt to win acceptance from peers: defying authority? (also in XIV)	−0.49	2.18	1.46
	15	How often is child tense and worried?	−0.48	2.99	1.18
	13j	How happy does child get when he hurts others?	−0.42	2.32	0.95

17h	How often does child show worry by doing work badly? (also in XIV)	−0.39	3.09	1.39
17g	How often does child show worry by getting silly?	−0.38	2.67	1.20
19c	How often does child show anger by throwing or breaking things?	−0.37	1.40	0.85
14g	How often does child show he's happy by settling down to work? (also in XIV)	+0.38	3.32	1.16
11b	Child does best work with group. (also in XIV)	+0.43	2.98	1.18
26	To what extent does discipline work with child, improve his behavior?	+0.46	2.89	1.10
27a	When you ask child to do something, to what extent will he do it immediately?	+0.48	3.33	1.21
7	When working at something he is interested in, how long does he keep at it?	+0.50	3.31	1.30
8	How long does child work at something he is not interested in? (also in XIV)	+0.56	2.14	1.34

II

Sociability

33a	In comparison to other children in class, rate child: leadership.	−0.79	2.62	1.39
22e	How often do other children choose him as helper, team member?	−0.77	2.36	1.27
22d	How often do other children choose him for leadership position? (also in XIV)	−0.75	2.00	1.21
33d	In comparison to other children in class rate child: physical co-ordination.	−0.75	3.22	1.23
10b	With other children, how much does child make friends?	−0.72	3.04	1.26
33c	In comparison to other children in class, rate child: ability to make friends.	−0.69	3.02	1.34
10a	With other children, how much does child go along with others?	−0.65	2.94	1.09
4	How good is child at athletics?	−0.64	3.24	1.10
22c	How often do other children praise him?	−0.64	2.24	1.17
33b	In comparison to other children in class, rate child: sociability.	−0.61	3.45	1.44
23f	How does child attempt to win acceptance from peers: directing, managing appropriate classroom activities? (also in XIV)	−0.54	2.00	1.30

Table 20. (Continued)

Factor Number	Question Number	Description	Loading	Mean	S.D.
II	9c	How often does child play with children his age outside the classroom? (also in VII)	−0.40	4.46	0.76
	12	How often is child happy?	−0.39	3.61	1.15
	9d	How often does child play with older children outside the classroom?	−0.37	2.44	1.21
	11c	Child does best work in front of class. (also in XIV)	−0.36	2.66	1.14
	17f	How often does child show worry by getting quiet?	+0.36	2.32	1.15
	24e	How does child attempt to win acceptance from teacher: Helplessness, dependency.	+0.43	2.22	1.43
	17e	How often does child show worry by going off by himself?	+0.47	2.49	1.17
	22a	How often do other children ignore him?	+0.48	2.31	1.40
	9a	How often does child play alone outside the classroom?	+0.56	2.36	1.29
III		*Dependency*			
	28e	Under what conditions does child come to you: when he wants affection?	−0.74	2.47	1.31
	28a	Under what conditions does child come to you: when needs assistance with schoolwork?	−0.65	3.21	1.10
	17i	How often child shows worry: come to you for comfort?	−0.63	2.14	1.11
	28d	Under what conditions does child come to you: when wants protection or reassurance?	−0.50	2.89	1.19
IV		*Sensitiveness*			
	16i	How upset does child get: when corrected or criticized?	+0.72	3.28	1.11
	16a	How upset does child get: when laughed at by adults?	+0.66	3.47	1.04
	16e	How upset does child get: when interrupted in some activity?	+0.61	2.80	1.14

Code	Question	r	Mean	SD
16j	How upset does child get: when feels promises have not been kept?	+0.60	3.78	0.76
16f	How upset does child get: when feels someone is unfair?	+0.55	4.01	0.94
16h	How upset does child get: when doesn't do as well as he wants?	+0.52	3.61	1.08
16b	How upset does child get: when laughed at by children? (also in VII)	+0.48	3.84	1.06
32g	If you refuse to do what he asks of you, he gets hurt and leaves.	+0.43	1.87	1.09

V Activity Level

Code	Question	r	Mean	SD
2b	How much does child talk on the playground?	+0.82	3.87	1.06
1a	How active is child in the classroom?	+0.81	3.68	1.25
3b	How noisy is child on the playground?	+0.78	3.60	1.14
2a	How much does child talk in the classroom?	+0.76	3.60	1.22
1b	How active is child on the playground?	+0.70	4.05	1.16
3a	How noisy is child in the classroom?	+0.68	3.20	1.34
23c	How does child attempt to win acceptance from peers: showing off, clowning?	+0.45	3.08	1.47
20a	How often does child bite his nails?	+0.44	1.36	0.88
16m	How upset does child get when he is alone?	+0.44	2.62	0.93
17d	How often does child show worry: gets fidgety?	+0.42	3.33	1.35
14h	How often does child show he is happy: is quiet?	−0.48	3.12	1.31

VI Resistance to Direction

Code	Question	r	Mean	SD
27d	When you ask child to do something, to what extent will he do it if you threaten him?	+0.79	2.94	1.33
27e	When you ask child to do something, to what extent will he do it if you promise activity he will enjoy?	+0.78	3.13	1.17
27f	When you ask child to do something, to what extent will he do it after being punished?	+0.67	2.80	1.20
27c	When you ask child to do something, to what extent will he do it after you urge him?	+0.65	3.13	1.15
9e	How often does child play with pets outside the classroom?	+0.43	2.96	0.94
20f	How often does child act ashamed?	+0.37	1.79	0.73

Table 20. (Continued)

Factor Number	Question Number	Description	Loading	Mean	S.D.
VII		*Manipulativeness*			
	31g	How often does child try to get things from you: says he has right to ask?	+0.54	1.66	1.06
	24d	How does child attempt win acceptance from teacher: flattery, charm	+0.50	1.55	0.89
	23e	How does child attempt win acceptance from peers: bribing with gifts, etc.?	+0.37	1.24	0.53
	31b	How often does child try to get things from you: suggest indirectly?	+0.37	2.12	0.97
	16b	How upset does child get when laughed at by children? (also in IV)	−0.38	3.84	1.06
	9c	How often does child play with children his age outside classroom? (also in II)	−0.47	4.46	0.76
VIII		*Immaturity*			
	9b	How often does child play with younger children outside classroom?	−0.73	1.75	1.13
	27g	When you ask child do something, to what extent will he absolutely refuse to do it?	−0.45	1.65	1.05
	5	How good is child at doing things with hands?	+0.38	3.13	0.95
IX		*Insecurity*			
	19d	How often does child show anger by crying?	−0.78	1.62	1.03
	17a	How often does child show worry by crying?	−0.77	1.54	0.96
	16k	How upset does child get when nobody pays attention to him? (also in IV)	−0.45	3.34	1.06
	11a	Child does best work: by himself.	+0.37	3.73	1.05
	16d	How upset does child get when punished physically?	+0.37	3.79	0.90

Destructiveness, Whininess

X				
17k	How often does child show worry by complaining something hurts him?	+0.78	1.61	0.98
21b	How often does child take things that don't belong to him?	+0.74	1.56	1.07
21d	How often does child tear up or break other people's things?	+0.73	1.39	0.77
21a	How often does child talk back to adults?	+0.73	1.87	1.27
20d	How often does child not feel well?	+0.67	1.52	0.85
17j	How often does child show worry by having temper tantrums?	+0.61	1.54	0.97
20e	How often does child say people don't like him?	+0.59	1.67	1.06
32c	If you refuse to do what he asks, he complains, cries.	+0.57	1.91	1.34
17b	How often does child show worry by whining and complaining?	+0.55	2.39	1.25
20c	How often does child show fear?	+0.43	1.61	1.02
13m	How happy does child get when breaking things?	+0.41	2.20	0.83
32a	If you refuse to do what he asks, he accepts your answer.	−0.61	3.56	1.15

Responsiveness to Positive Reward

XI				
13e	How happy does child get when he has time with you?	−0.74	3.87	0.92
13a	How happy does child get when he is praised?	−0.70	4.34	0.89
13b	How happy does child get when he gets presents? (also in VI)	−0.61	3.93	0.74
13c	How happy does child get when he gets affection?	−0.54	4.04	0.85
11d	Child does best work with teacher. (also in XV)	−0.47	3.69	0.94
13g	How happy does child get when taken on trips and outings?	−0.43	3.88	0.84
31a	How often does child try to get things from you by asking you directly for what he wants?	−0.36	3.39	1.02

Expressions of Happiness

XII				
14c	How often does child show he is happy: chatter and talks?	−0.70	4.05	0.99
14d	How often does child show he is happy: gets excited?	−0.67	3.58	1.17
14a	How often does child show he is happy: laughs out loud?	−0.67	3.42	1.20
14f	How often does child show he is happy: clowns, plays around?	−0.62	3.24	1.22
14e	How often does child show he is happy: shows affection?	−0.52	2.82	1.14
14b	How often does child show he is happy: whistles, sings?	−0.49	2.46	1.09
23b	How does child attempt to win acceptance from peers: laughing joking?	−0.46	3.25	1.34

Table 20. (Continued)

Factor Number	Question Number	Description	Loading	Mean	S.D.
XIII		*Dexterity*			
	13h	How happy does he get when doing things by himself?	−0.64	2.80	0.83
	5	How good is child at doing things with hands?	−0.55	3.13	0.95
	13n	How happy does he get when taking things apart?	−0.52	2.86	0.90
	33f	In comparison to other children in class, rate child: work with hands.	−0.49	2.92	1.01
XIV		*Interpersonal Effectiveness*			
	24a	How does child attempt to win acceptance from teacher: completing all required tasks.	−0.73	2.98	1.39
	33e	In comparison with other children in class, rate child: schoolwork.	−0.67	2.74	1.27
	23a	How does child attempt to win acceptance from peers: helping others.	−0.62	2.48	1.31
	16l	How upset does child get when somebody else gets hurt?	−0.61	2.64	0.95
	24b	How does child attempt to win acceptance from peers: offering help.	−0.55	3.14	1.41
	27a	When you ask child to do something, to what extent will he do it immediately.	−0.53	3.33	1.21
	14g	How often does child show he is happy: settles down to work? (also in I)	−0.53	3.32	1.16
	27h	When you ask child to do something, to what extent will he remember to do it next time on his own? (also in II)	−0.51	2.59	1.40

No.	Item			
30	How well does this child communicate ideas?	−0.51	3.40	1.31
11b	Child does best work: with group. (also in I)	−0.50	2.98	1.18
26	To what extent does discipline work with child, improve his behavior? (also in I)	−0.46	2.90	1.19
24f	How does child attempt to win acceptance from teacher: performing extra?	−0.45	2.42	1.24
27b	When you ask child to do something, to what extent will he do it later, without urging?	−0.44	2.40	1.18
131	How happy does child get when he knows he has done something well?	−0.44	4.33	0.73
31d	How often does child try to get things from you: is especially "good"?	−0.43	2.66	1.24
31f	How often does child try to get things from you: show you good objective reasons for what he wants?	−0.42	2.46	1.05
8	How long does child work at something he is not interested in? (also in I)	−0.41	2.14	1.34
13i	How happy does child get when he helps others?	−0.41	3.38	0.94
13d	How happy does child get when he is given responsibility? (also in XI)	−0.38	3.93	1.14
29	How well does child communicate his feelings? (also in II)	−0.36	3.21	1.33
28b	Under what conditions does he come to you: when he has done something wrong?	−0.35	1.74	0.91
17h	How often does child show worry: does his work badly? (also in I)	+0.59	3.09	1.39
23h	How does child attempt to win acceptance from peers: defying authority? (I)	+0.44	2.18	1.46

Table 21. Observers' Ratings of School Behavior: Referred and Nonreferred Children

	Referred		Nonreferred		
	X	S.E. X	X	S.E. X	Nonreferred-Referred
Playground (peers)					
Negative Social Impact	5.00[a]	0.31	3.60	0.24	−1.40**
Positive Social Impact	4.48	0.30	3.65	0.47	−0.83(*)
Class (teacher)					
Negative Social Impact	4.47	0.24	3.48	0.18	−0.99**
Positive Social Impact	3.60	0.27	3.48	0.40	−0.12
Class (peers)					
Negative Social Impact	4.30	0.21	4.01	0.36	−0.29
Positive Social Impact	3.21	0.24	3.41	0.41	+0.20

[a] scores represent mean C-scores of the adjectives contained within the Negative and Positive Impact factors (C-scores computed with respect to a random sample of children).

(*) $p = .20$.
** $p = .01$.

Table 22. Observers' Ratings of School Behavior in Terms of Referral Category

	Predominant Referral Category			
	Aggression	Hyper-activity	Social Withdrawal	Attention Control
Negative Social Impact Classroom				
Child-teacher	5.46	5.38	4.46	4.44
Child-peers	5.36	5.27	4.77	4.45
N	23[a]	15	17	34
Playground	3.71	3.57	4.26	4.47
N	19	15	17	30
Positive Social Impact Classroom				
Child-teacher	4.43	5.19	4.89	4.44
Child peers	4.82	4.73	5.11	4.41
N	23	15	17	34
Playground	5.50	4.75	4.41	4.41
N	19	15	17	30

[a] Children observed in the classroom were not always on the playground when observations were scheduled. The N for these two settings therefore varies slightly.

Table 23. Formal Characteristics of Clinicians and Treatments by Year

		Cases by Sex of Therapist		Cases by experience level		Total N Clinic Contracts	Mean N Total Clinic Contracts	Cases in for Follow-Up	M[c]	C[d]	D[e]
		M	F	X[a]	NX[b]						
Information Feedback											
Year I	N	11	4	9	6	149	9.9	12	5	18	1
	%	73	27	60	40						
Year II	N	12	3	10	5	106	7.1	7	5		1
	%	80	20	67	33						
Total	N	23	7	19	11	255	8.5	19	10	7	2
	%	(76)	(23)	(67)	(33)			(63)			(7)
Parent Counseling											
Year I	N	4	7	—	11	63	5.7	7	5	6	2
	%	36	64		100						
Year II	N	4	13	17	—	100	5.9	12	7	9	3
	%	24	76	100							
Total	N	8	20	17	11	163	5.8	19	12	15	5
	%	(29)	(71)					(70)			
Child Therapy											
Year I	N	—	17	17	—	212	12.5	10	9	20	7
	%		100	100							(21)
Year II	N	8	8	15	1	199	12.0	10	19	20	—
	%	50	50	94	6						
Total	N	8	25	32	1	411	12.2	20	28	40	7
	%	(24)	(76)	(94)	(3)			(61)			

[a] Experienced clinician.
[b] Not experienced clinician.
[c] Missed appointments.
[d] Cancelled appointments.
[e] Dropped out of treatment.

Table 24. Teacher Inventory: Prepost Differences in Factor Scores

| Factor | Pretreatment–Second Follow-Up | | | |
	Information Feedback	Child Therapy	Parent Counseling	Nonreferred
1. Interpersonal conflict	—.23*	—.17	—.22	—.03
2. Sociability	.09	—.07	.04	—.19
3. Dependency on teacher	—.12	—.11	—.11	—.34*
4. Sensitive—suspicious	—.38*	—.28	—.27	—.29*
5. Activity level	—.21	—.28	—.32*	—.24*
6. Resists direction	—.22	—.26	—.09	—.25
7. Manipulative	—.01	0	.16	.02
8. Immaturity	—.24	.02	0	.01
9. Crying, seeks attention	—.21	—.15	—.11	—.02
10. General protest	—.18	—.11	—.16	—.02
11. Depends on positive reward	—.40*	—.08	—.24	—.28
12. Expresses happiness	—.10	—.24	—.02	—.24
13. Physical dexterity	.31*	.09	.10	—.27
14. Interpersonal effectiveness	.12	.17	—.03	—.15
N	19	12	11	17

Note 1: In 11 of the 14 factors, the original–second follow-up difference for Information Feedback the largest difference of the three intervention groups.

Note 2: four of the 14 differences in the feedback group are at or near the $p < .05$ level. There are *no* significant differences for the Therapy group, and only one difference for the Parent Counseling group.

Table 25. Family Member Ratings of TV Excerpts. Rater Effects

Analysis of Variance	IB: Negative Social Impact		IIB: Positive Social Impact	
Father is rater				
Group (R, NR)	NR $<$ R[a]	.10[b]		
Family member				
rated (F, M, C)	M $<$ F $<$ C	.01		
Group by				
member rated	R: M $<$ F $<$ C	.01		
	NR: F $=$ M $=$ C			
Mother is rater				
Group (R, NR)			NR $>$ R	.01
Family member				
rated (F, M, C)			F $=$ C $>$ M	.05
Group by				
member rated				
Child is rater				
Group (R, NR)				
Family member				
rated (F, M, C)	M $=$ F $<$ C	.01		
Group by				
member rated				

[a] The symbol $<$ indicates that the mean for the first group is smaller than the mean for the second group; $>$ indicates that the first mean is larger than the second.

[b] significance level of the comparisons.

Table 26.   Family Member Ratings of TV Excerpts. Person Rated Effects

Analysis of Variance	IB: Negative Social Impact		IIB: Positive Social Impact	
Ratings of father				
Group (R, NR)	NR < R[a]	.01[b]	NR > R	.001
Rater (F, M, C)	C > M > F	.10		
G × R				
Ratings of mother				
Group (R, NR)				
Rater (F, M, C)			F = C > M	.05
G × R				
Ratings of child				
Group (R, NR)	NR < R	.001	NR > R	.10
Rater (F, M, C)				
G × R				

[a] The symbol < indicates that the mean for the first group is smaller than the mean for the second group; > indicates that the first mean is larger than the second.
[b] Significance level of the comparisons.

Table 27.   Family Member Ratings of TV Excerpts. TV Family Adjective Ratings Anova: R — NR and SEL:[a] Person Rating (Fa, Mo, Ch): Rater Effects

	IB: Negative Social Impact				IIB: Positive Social Impact		
	df	MS	F	p<	MS	F	p<
Father is rating							
Group (R-NR)	1	29.25	3.95	.10	10.79	2.10	
Person rated (R)	2	7.70	5.40	.01	1.30	1.24	
G × R	2	7.56	5.30	.01	0.78	0.74	
Error	96	3.42			2.41		
Mother is Rating							
Group (R-NR)	1	14.80	3.18		14.74	6.27	.01
Person rated (R)	2	0.45	0.28		4.72	4.64	.05
G × R	2	1.72	1.06		0.43	0.43	
Error	102	2.64			1.46		
Child is Rating							
Group (R-NR)	1	6.21	0.98		18.63	2.99	
Person rated (R)	2	5.46	6.32	.01	0.06	0.09	
G × R	2	0.85	0.98		1.05	1.66	
Error	96	2.69			2.50		

[a] Since there were no significant socioeconomic level results, these data are not reported.

Table 28. TV FARS ANOVA: R — NR and SEL. Person Being Rated (Fa, Mo, Ch)

		IB: Negative Social Impact			IIB: Positive Social Impact		
	df	MS	F	$p<$	MS	F	$p<$
Father is rated							
R-NR:							
Group	1	21.03	7.37	.01	33.51	15.79	.001
Rater	2	6.98	2.45	.10	2.96		
G × R	2	0.45			0.05		
Error	127	2.85			2.12		
SEL:							
Group	2	3.09			2.79		
Rater	2	2.56			1.23		
G × R	2	2.35			2.35		
Error	124	2.97			2.33		
Mother is rated							
R-NR:							
Group	1	1.31			2.71		
Rater	2	2.68			6.49	3.40	.05
G × R	2	0.03			0.04		
Error	136	2.22			1.91		
SEL:							
Group	2	1.10			1.83		
Rater	2	1.78			5.72	2.98	.10
G × R	4	1.26			1.17		
Error	133	2.24			1.92		
Child is rated							
R-NR:							
Group	1	52.77	19.13	.001	17.43	8.91	
Rater	2	4.15			0.51		
G × R	2	3.93			0.11		
Error	141	2.76			1.96		
SEL:							
Group	2	10.52	3.51	.05	6.38	3.21	.05
Rater	2	0.70			0.02		
G × R	4	4.03			2.24		
Error	138	2.99			1.99		

Table 29. Affective Lability Changes: ANOVA Summary for Fathers

Source	Evaluative Range F	df	Positive Extreme F	df	Negative Extreme F	df
Group[a]	9.02*	1,5	1.20	1,5	0.14	1,5
Period[b]	1.99	1,5	0.91	1,5	3.98	1,5
Time[c]	13.07*	1,5	6.19(*)	1,5	1.15	1,5
Time × period	0.00	1,5	1.88	1,5	2.38	1,5
Group × period	0.03	1,5	0.89	1,5	1.68	1,5
Group × time	4.83(*)	1,5	0.55	1,5	8.67*	1,5
Group × Time × period	0.48	1,5	0.37	1,5	0.22	1,5

[a] Feedback versus other treatment.
[b] Free interaction versus problem definition.
[c] Original versus follow-up.
(*) $p = .10$.
* $p < .05$.

Table 30. Affective Lability Changes: ANOVA Summary for Children

Source	Evaluative Range F	df	Positive Extreme F	df	Negative Extreme F	df
Group	2.65	1,8	0.00	1,8	3.62	1,8
Period	2.47	1,8	1.29	1,8	7.50*	1,8
Time	5.71*	1,8	0.01	1,8	5.33*	1,8
Time × period	3.80	1,8	3.07	1,8	9.56*	1,8
Group × period	2.64	1,8	0.00	1,8	3.71	1,8
Group × time	9.23*	1,8	5.84*	1,8	0.20	1,8
Group × time × period	6.95*	1,8	1.07	1,8	11.15**	1,8

* $p < .05$.
** $p < .01$.

References

Alkire, A. A. Social power and accuracy of communication in families of disturbed and non disturbed preadolescents. Unpublished doctoral dissertation, University of California, Los Angeles, 1967.

Alkire, A. A. Social power and communication within families of disturbed and non disturbed preadolescents. *Journal of Personality and Social Psychology*, 1969, **13**, 335–349.

Alkire, A. A. Enactment of social power and role behavior in families of disturbed and nondisturbed preadolescents. *Developmental Psychology*, 1972, **7** (2).

Alkire, A. A., Collum, M. E., Kaswan, J., and Love, L. Information exchange and accuracy of verbal communication under social power conditions. *Journal of Personality and Social Psychology*, 1968, **9**, 301–308.

Ammons, R. B. and Huth, R. W. The full-range picture vocabulary test. I. Preliminary scale. *Journal of Psychology*, 1949, **28**, 51–64.

Anderson, N. H. Averaging versus adding as a stimulus-combination rule in impression formation. *Journal of Experimental Psychology*, 1965, **70**, 394–400.

Bandura, A. and Walters, R. H. *Adolescent aggression*. New York: Ronald Press, 1959.

Baratz, S. S. and Baratz, J. Early childhood interventions: The social science base of institutional racism. *Harvard Educational Review*, 1970, **40**, 29–50.

Barker, R. G. On the nature of the environment. *Journal of Social Issues*, 1963, **19**, 17–83.

Bateson, G., Jackson, D. D., Haley, J., and Weakland, J. Toward a theory of schizophrenia. *Behavioral Science*, 1956, **1**, 251–264.

Baum, O., Felzer S., D'Zonura T., and Shumaker, E. Psyhotherapy, dropouts, lower socio-economic patients. *American Journal of Orthopsychiatry*, 1966, **36**, 629–635.

Beakel, N. G. and Mehrabian, A. Inconsistent communications and psychopathology. *Journal of Abnormal Psychology*, 1969, **74**, 126–130.

Becker, W. C. Consequences of different kinds of parental discipline. In J. L. Hoffman and L. W. Hoffman (Eds.), *Review of child development research*, Vol. I. New York: Russell Sage Foundation, 1964.

Becker, W. C., Peterson, D. R., Hellmer, L. A., Shoemaker, D. F., and Quay, H. C. Factors in parental behavior and personality as related to problem behavior in children. *Journal of Consulting Psychology*, 1959, **23**, 107–118.

Bellak, L. and Small, L. *Emergency psychotherapy and brief psychotherapy*. New York: Grune and Stratton, 1965.

Bennis, W. G., Schein, E. H., Stelle F. I., and Berlew, D. E. (Eds.) *Interpersonal dynamics: Essays and readings on human interaction*. Homewood, Ill.: The Dorsey Press, 1968.

Benson, L. *Fatherhood: a sociological perspective.* New York: Random House, 1968.

Betz, B. Studies of the therapist's role in the treatment of the schizophrenic patient. *American Journal of Psychiatry,* 1967, **123**, 963–971.

Blood, R. O. and Wolfe, D. K. *Husbands and wives: the dynamics of married living.* New York: The Free Press, 1960.

Bodin, A. M. Family interaction: a social-clinical study of synthetic, normal and problem family triads. In W. D. Winter and A. J. Ferreira (Eds.), *Family interaction: readings and commentary. Palo Alto, Calif.: Science and Behavior Books,* 1969.

Brehm, J. W. *A theory of psychological reactance.* New York: Academic Press, 1966.

Bronfenbrenner, A. Child relationships in a social context. In J. C. Glidewell (Ed.), *Parental attitudes and child behavior.* Springfield, Ill.: Charles C. Thomas, 1961.

Brookover, W. B., Erickson, E., Hamacheck, D., Joiner, L., Lepere, J., Peterson, A., and Thomas S. Self-concept of ability and school achievement. In L. Gorlow and W. Katkovski (Eds.), *Readings in the psychology of adjustment* (2nd ed.). New York: McGraw-Hill, 1968.

Bugental, D. E., Kaswan, J. W., and Love, L. R. Perception of contradictory meanings conveyed by verbal and nonverbal channels. *Journal of Personality and Social Psychology,* 1970, **16**, 647–655.

Bugental, D. E., Kaswan, J. W., Love, L. R., and Fox, M. N. Child versus adult perception of evaluative messages in verbal, vocal, and visual channels. *Developmental Psychology,* 1970, **2**, 367–375.

Bugental, D. E., Love, L. R., and Gianeto, R. M. Perfidious feminine faces. *Journal of Personality and Social Psychology,* 1971, **17**, 314–318.

Bugental, D. E., Love, L. R., and Kaswan, J. W. Videotaped family interaction: differences reflecting presence and type of child disturbance. *Journal of Abnormal Psychology,* 1972, **79**(3), 285–290.

Bugental, D. E., Love, L. R., Kaswan, J. W., and April, C. Verbal-nonverbal conflict in parental messages to normal and disturbed children. *Journal of Abnormal Psychology,* 1971, **77**, 6–10.

Caplan, G. General introduction and over-view. In G. Caplan (Ed.), *Prevention of mental disorders in children.* New York: Basic Books, 1961, pp. 3–30.

Caputo, D. V. The parents of the schizophrenic. *Family Process,* 1963, **2**, 339–356.

Carkhuff, R. R. Differential function of lay and professional helpers. *Journal of Counseling Psychology,* 1968, **15**, 117–126.

Cartwright, R. D. Psychotherapeutic processes. *Annual Reviews of Psychology,* **19**. Palo Alto, Calif.: 1968.

Cartwright, R. D. and Vogel, J. L. A comparison of changes in psychoneurotic patients during matched period of therapy and no-therapy. *Journal of Consulting Psychology,* 1960, **24**, 121–127.

Cole, M., Gay, J., Glick, J. A., and Sharp, D. W. *The cultural context of learning and thinking.* New York: Basic Books, 1971.

Cowen, E. L., Huser, J., Beach, D. R., and Rappaport, J. Parental perceptions of young children and their relation to indexes of adjustment. *Journal of Consulting and Clinical Psychology,* 1970, **34**(1), 97–103.

Crandall, V., Dewey, R., Katkovsky, W., and Preston, A. Parents' attitudes and behaviors and grade-school children's academic achievements. *Journal of Genetic Psychology,* 1964, **104**, 53–66.

Dember, W. N. *The psychology of perception.* New York: Holt, Rinehart and Winston, 1960.

Deutsch, M. Some psychosocial aspects of learning in the disadvantaged. In Martin Deutsch (Ed.), *The disadvantaged child.* New York: Basic Books, 1967.

Dickinson, T. C., Neubert, J., and McDermott, D. Relationship of scores on the Full Range Picture Vocabulary Test and the Wechsler Adult Intelligence Scale in a vocational rehabilitation setting. *Psychological Reports,* 1968, **83**, 1263–1266.

Eiduson, B. Retreat from help. *American Journal of Orthopsychiatry,* 1968, **38**, 910–921.

English, O. S. The psychological role of the father in the family. *Social Casework,* **35**, 329.

Epstein, N. Priorities for change—some preliminary proposals from the White House Conference on children. *Children,* 1971, **18**, 2–7.

Eysenck, H. J. The effects of psychotherapy. *International Journal of Psychiatry,* 1965, **1**, 97–178.

Farina, A. Patterns of role dominance and conflict in parents of schizophrenic patients. *Journal of Abnormal and Social Psychology,* 1960, **61**, 31–38.

Ferreira, A. J. and Winter, W. D. Family interaction and decision-making. *Archives of General Psychiatry,* 1965, **13**, 214–223.

Festinger, L. *The theory of cognitive dissonance.* New York: Harper and Row, 1957.

Final Report of Joint Commission on Mental Health of Children, Inc. *Digest of crisis in child mental health: Challenge for the 1970's.* Washington, D.C.: Joint Commission on Mental Health Children, Inc., 1969.

Fontana, A. F. Familial etiology of schizophrenia: Is a scientific methodology possible? *Psychological Bulletin,* 1966, **66**, 214–227.

Ford, D. H. and Urban, H. B. *Systems of psychotherapy.* New York: Wiley, 1963.

Ford, D. H. and Urban, H. B. Psychotherapy. In *Annual Reviews of Psychology,* **18**. Palo Alto, Calif.: 1967.

Frank, J. D. *Persuasion and healing.* Baltimore: Johns Hopkins Press, 1961.

Frank, J. D., Nash, E. H., Stone, A. R., and Imber, S. D. Immediate and long-term symptomatic course of psychiatric outpatients. *American Journal of Psychiatry,* 1963, **120**, 429–439.

Frank, G. H. The role of the family in the development of psychopathology. *Psychological Bulletin,* 1965, **64**, 191–205.

French, J. R. P. Jr., and Raven, B. H. The basis of social power. In D. Cartwright (Ed.), *Studies in social power.* Ann Arbor: University of Michigan Press, 1959.

Garner, W. *Uncertainty and structure as psychological concepts.* New York: Wiley, 1962.

Gibson, J. J. *The senses considered as perceptual systems.* New York: Houghton Mifflin, 1966.

Gibson, J. J. and Gibson, E. Perceptual learning: Differentiation or enrichment? *Psychological Review,* 1955, **62**, 32–41.

Glasser, W. *Reality therapy: A new approach to psychiatry.* New York: Harper & Row, 1965.

Glueck, S. and Glueck, E. *Unraveling juvenile delinquency*. Cambridge: Harvard University Press, 1950.

Goin, M. K., Yamamoto, J., and Silverman, J. Therapy congruent with class-linked expectations. *General Psychiatry*, 1965, **13**, 133–137.

Goodstein, L. D. and Rowley, W. N. A further study of MMPI differences between parents of disturbed and nondisturbed children. *Journal of Consulting Psychology*, 1961, **25**, 460.

Gould, R. Dr. Strangeclass: or how I stopped worrying about the theory and began treating the blue-collar worker. *American Journal of Orthopsychiatry*, 1967, **37**, 78–86.

Haggard, E. A., Brekstad, A., and Skard. A. On the reliability of the anamnestic interview. *Journal of Abnormal and Social Psychology*, 1960, **61**, 311–318.

Haley, J. Research on family patterns: an instrument measure. *Family Process*, 1964, **3**, 41–65.

Hartman, H. *Essays on ego psychology*. New York: International University Press, 1964.

Hays, W. L. *Statistics for psychologists*. New York: Holt, Rinehart & Winston, 1963.

Heider, F. *The psychology of interpersonal relations*. New York: Wiley, 1958.

Heinecke, C. M. and Goldman, A. Research on psychotherapy with children: a review and suggestion for further study. *American Journal of Orthopsychiatry*, 1960, **30**, 483–494.

Hetherington, E. M. A developmental study of the effects of sex of the dominant parent on sex-role preference, identification and imitation in children. *Journal of Personality and Social Psychology*, 1965, **2**, 188–194.

Hetherington, E. M. and Prautie, G. Effects of the parental dominance, warmth, and conflict on imitation in children. *Journal of Personality and Social Psychology*, 1967, **6**, 119–125.

Hoffman, L. W. and Lippett, R. The measurement of family life variables. In P. H. Mussen (Ed.), *Handbook of research methods in child development*. New York: Wiley, 1960.

Hoffman, M. L. Power assertion by the parent and its impact on the child. *Child Development*, 1960, **31**, 129–143.

Hollingshead, A. B. and Redlich, R. C. *Social class and mental illness: a community study*. New York: Wiley, 1958.

Howe, E. S. and Silverstein, A. B. Comparison of two short-form derivatives of the Taylor Manifest Anxiety Scale. *Psychological Reports*. 1960, **6**, 9–10.

Hunt, R. Occupational status and the disposition of cases in a child guidance clinic. *International Journal of Social Psychiatry*, 1962, **8**, 199–210.

Hutchinson. J. G. Family interaction patterns and the emotionally disturbed child. In W. D. Winter and A. J. Ferreira, (Eds.), *Family interaction: readings and commentary*. Palo Alto, Calif.: Science and Behavior Books, 1969.

Hyman, R. and Berger, L. The effects of psychotherapy: discussion. *International Journal of Psychiatry*, 1965, **1**, 317–322.

Jackson, D. D. and Weakland, J. Conjoint family therapy: some considerations on theory, technique, and results. *Psychiatry*, 1961, **24**, 30–45.

Jones, E. E. and Davis, K. E. From acts to dispositions: the attribution process in person perception. In Leonard Berkowitz (Ed.), *Advances in experimental social psychology*, Vol. 2. New York: Academic Press, 1965.

Kagan, J. Acquisition and significance of sex typing and sex role identity. In M. L. Hoffman and L. W. Hoffman (Eds.), *Review of child development research*. New York: Russell Sage, 1964.

Kaplan, M. F. How response dispositions integrate with stimulus information. *Technical Report No. 19*. La Jolla, Calif.: Center for Human Information Processing, 1971.

Kaswan, J. W. and Love, L. R. Confrontation as a method of clinical intervention. *Journal of Nervous and Mental Diseases*, 1969, **148**, 224–237.

Kaswan, J. W., Love, L. R., and Rodnick, E. H. Information feedback as a method of clinical intervention and consultation. In C. Spielberger (Ed.), *Current topics in clinical and community psychology*, Vol. 3. New York: Academic Press, 1971.

Kaswan, J. W., Love, L. R., Seeman, A., and Overman, B. School behavior ratings of "disturbed" and "normal" children as a function of socioeconomic level. Unpublished manuscript, University of California, Los Angeles, 1967.

Kaswan, J. W., Young, S., and Nakamura, C. Y. Stimulus determinants of choice behavior in visual pattern discrimination. *Journal of Experimental Psychology*, 1965, **69**, 441–449.

Kelley, H. H. Attribution theory in social psychology. In D. Levine (Ed.), *Nebraska symposium on motivation*. Lincoln, Neb.: University of Nebraska Press, 1967, pp. 192–238.

Kelly, J. Ecological constraints on mental health services. *American Psychologist*, 1966, **21**, 535–539.

Kiesler, D. J. Some myths of psychotherapy research and the search for a paradigm. *Psychological Bulletin*, 1966, **65**, 110–136.

King, B. T. and Janis, T. L. Comparison of effectiveness of improvised versus non-improvised role-playing in producing opinion changes. *Human Relations*, 1956, **9**, 177–186.

Klein, G. S. The Menninger Foundation research on perception and personality, 1947–1952: a review. *Bulletin of the Menninger Clinic*, 1953, **7**, 93–99.

Knapp, R. H. and Holzberg, J. D. Characteristics of college students volunteering for service to mental patients. *Journal of Consulting Psychology*, 1964, **28**, 82–85.

Krauss, R. M. and Glucksberg, S. Some aspects of verbal communication in children. A paper presented in the symposium *Approaches to Interpersonal Communication* at the American Psychological Association meeting in Chicago, Ill., Sept., 1965.

Labov, W. The logic of non-standard English. In F. William (Ed.), *Language and poetry*. Chicago: Markham, 1970.

Leacock, E. B., Teaching and learning in city schools. New York: Basic Books, 1969.

Leary, T. *Interpersonal diagnosis of personality*. New York: Ronald Press, 1957.

Le Masters, E. E. Parents in modern America: a sociological analysis. Homewood, Ill.: Dorsey Press, 1970.

Lennard, H. L. and Bernstein, A. *Patterns in human interaction*. San Francisco: Jossey, Bass, 1969.

Lenneberg, E. H. Language, evaluation and purposive behavior. In S. Diamond (Ed.), *Culture in history: essays in honor of Paul Radin*. New York: 1960.

Levinger, G. Supplementary methods in family research. *Family Process*, 1963, **2**, 357–366.

Levitt, E. E. The results of psychotherapy with children: an evaluation. *Journal of Consulting Pscyhology*, 1957, **21**, 189–196.

Levitt, E. E. Psychotherapy with children: a further evaluation. *Behavior Research and Therapy*, 1963, **1**, 45–51.

Levitt, E. E. Reply to Hood-Williams. *Journal of Consulting Psychology*, 1966, **24**, 89–91.

Levy, D. M. Maternal overprotection. New York: Columbia University Press, 1943.

Lewin, K. Group decision and social change. In T. M. Newcomb and E. L. Hartley (Eds.), *Readings in social psychology*. New York: Holt, Rinehart & Winston, 1947, pp. 330–344.

Lidz, T. *The person*. New York: Basic Books, 1968.

Lidz, T., Parker, B., and Cornelison, A. The role of the father in the family environment of the schizophrenic patient. *American Journal of Psychiatry*, 1956, **113**, 126–132.

Liverant, Shephard. MMPI differences between parents of disturbed and nondisturbed children. *Journal of Consulting Psychology*, 1959, **23**, 256–260.

Love, L. R., Kaswan, J. K., and Bugental, D. E. Differential effectiveness of three clinical interventions for different socioeconomic groupings. *Journal of Consulting and Clinical Psychology*, 1972, **39**, 347–360.

Lowry, L. G. (Ed.) *Orthopsychiatry, 1923—1948: retrospect and prospect*. New York: American Orthopsychiatric Association, 1948.

Maas, H. S., Kahan, A. J., Stein, H. D., and Summer, D. Sociocultural factors in psychiatric clinic services for children. *Smith College Studies of Social Work*, 1955, **25**, 1–90.

McCord, W., McCord, J., and Howard, A. Familial correlates of aggression in non-delinquent male children. *Journal of Abnormal and Social Psychology*, 1961, **62**, 79–83.

McDermott, J. F., Harrison, S. I., Schrager, J., and Wilson, P. Social class and mental illness in children: observation of blue-collar families. *American Journal of Orthopsychiatry*, 1965, **35**(3), 500–508.

McGuire, W. J. The nature of attitudes and attitude change. In G. Lindzey and E. Aronson (Eds.) *Handbook of social psychology*, Vol. 3. Reading, Mass.: Addison-Wesley, 1969.

McNair, D. M. and Lorr, M. An analysis of professed psychotherapeutic techniques. *Journal of Consulting Psychology*, 1964, **28**, 265–271.

Merrill, B. A. A measurement of mother-child interaction. *Journal of Abnormal and Social Psychology*, 1946, **41**, 37–49.

Miller, G. A. The magical number seven, plus or minus two. *Psychological Review*, 1956, **63**, 81–97.

Mishler, E. G. and Waxler, N. E. *Interaction in families*. New York: Wiley, 1968.

Moustakas, C. E., Siegel, I. E., and Schalock, H. D. An objective method for the measurement and analysis of child-adult interaction. *Child Development*, 1956, **27**, 109–134.

Murrell, S. A. and Stachowiak, J. G. Consistency, rigidity, and power in the interaction of clinic and non-clinic families. *Journal of Abnormal Psychology,* 1967, **72,** 265–272.

Newcomb, T., Turner, R. H., and Converse, P. E. *Social psychology.* New York: Holt, Rinehart & Winston, 1965.

Osgood, C. E. Studies on the generality of affective meaning systems. *American Psychologist,* 1962, **17,** 10–28.

Osgood, C. E., Suci, C. J., and Tannenbaum, P. H. *The measurement of meaning.* Urbana: University of Illinois Press, 1957.

Osgood, C. E. and Tannenbaum, P. H. The principle of congruity in the prediction of attitude change. *Psychological Review,* 1955, **62,** 40–55.

Parsons, T. and Bales, R. F. (Eds.). *Family, socialization and interaction process.* Glencoe, Ill.: Free Press, 1955.

Paul, G. L. *Insight versus desensitization in psychotherapy: an experiment in anxiety reduction.* Palo Alto, Calif. Stanford University Press, 1966.

Paul, G. L. Strategy of outcome research in psychotherapy. *Journal of Consulting Psychology,* 1967, **31,** 109–118.

Peterson, D. R., Becker, W. C., Hellmer, L. A., Shoemaker, D. J., and Quay, H. C. Parental attitudes and child adjustment. *Child Development,* 1959, **30,** 119–130.

Peterson, D. R., Quay, H. C., and Tiffany, T. C. Personality factors related to juvenile delinquency. *Child Development,* 1961, **32,** 355–372.

Pollack, O. *Intergrating sociological and psychoanalytic concepts: an exploration in child psychotherapy.* New York: Russell Sage, 1956.

Poser, E. The effect of therapists' training on group therapeutic outcome. *Journal of Consulting Psychology,* 1966, **30,** 282–290.

Quay, H. C. and Quay, L. C. Behavior problems in early adolescence. *Child Development,* 1965, **36,** 215–220.

Rabbie, J M. Differential preference for companionship under threat. *Journal of Abnormal and Social Psychology,* 1963, **67,** 643–648.

Rapapport, D. The structure of psychoanalytic theory. *Psychological Issues,* 1960, **2**(2).

Raven, B. Social influence and power. In I. D. Steiner and M. Fishbein (Eds.), *Readings in contemporary social psychology.* New York: Holt, Rinehart & Winston, 1965.

Robbins, L. C. The accuracy of parental recall of aspects of child development and of child rearing practices. *Journal of Abnormal and Social Psychology,* 1963, **66,** 261–270.

Rogers, R., Gendlin, G. T., Kiesler, D. V., and Truax, C. B. *The therapeutic relationship and its impact: A study of psychotherapy with schizophrenics.* Madison: University of Wisconsin Press, 1967.

Rosenthal, R. and Jacobson, L. Teachers' expectations: Determinants of pupils' IQ gains. *Psychological Report,* 1966, **19,** 115–118.

Ross, A. C. Poor school achievement: A psychiatric study and classification. *Clinical Pediatrics,* 1966, **5,** 109.

Ross, A. O., and Lacey, H. M. Characteristics of terminators and remainers in child guidance treatment. *Journal of Consulting Pscyhology,* 1961, **25,** 420–424.

Sager, C. J., Masters, Y. J., Ronall, R. E., and Normand, W. C. Selection and engagement of patients in family therapy. *American Journal of Orthopsychiatry*, 1968, **38**, 715–723.

Sarason, S. B., Levine, M., Goldenberg, I. I., Cherlin, D. L., and Bennett, L. M. *Psychology in community settings.* New York: Wiley 1966.

Schachter, S. *The psychology of affiliation.* Stanford, Calif.: Stanford University Press, 1959.

Schaefer, E. S. A configuration analysis of children's reports of parent behavior. *Journal of Consulting Psychology*, 1965, **29**, 552–557.

Schofield, W. *Psychotherapy: the purchase of friendship.* Englewood Cliffs, N.J.: Prentice-Hall, 1964.

Schuham, A. I. The double-bind hypothesis a decade later. *Psychological Bulletin*, 1968, **68**, 409–416.

Schulman, R. E., Shoemaker, D. J., and Moelis, I. Laboratory measurement of parental behavior. *Journal of Consulting Pscyhology*, 1962, **26**, 109–114.

Schutz, W. C. *FIRO: a three-dimensional theory of interpersonal behavior.* New York: Rinehart, 1958.

Sears, R. R., Whiting, J. W. M., Nowlis, F., and Sears, P. S. Some child-rearing antecedents of aggression and dependency in young children. *Genetic Psychology Monographs*, 1953, **47**, 135–236.

Seeman, J., Barry, E., and Ellinwood, C. Interpersonal assessment of play therapy outcome. *Psychotherapy: Theory, Research and Practice*, 1964, **1**(2), 64–66.

Segall, M. H., Campbell, D. T., and Herskovitz, M. D. *The influence of culture on visual perception.* Indianapolis: Bobbs-Merrill, 1966.

Shapiro, J. G. Relationships between expert and neophyte ratings of therapeutic conditions. *Journal of Consulting and Clinical Psychology*, 1968, **32**, 87–89.

Siegelman, M. Evaluation of Bronfenbrenner's questionnaire for children concerning parental behavior. *Child Development*, 1965, **36**, 164–174.

Silberman, C. E. *Crisis in the classroom.* New York: Random House, 1970.

Solley, C. M. and Murphy, G. *The development of the perceptual world.* New York: Basic Books, 1960.

Speer, D. C. Behavior problem checklist (Peterson-Quay). *Journal of Consulting and Clinical Psychology*, 1971, **36**, 221–228.

Speer, D. C., Fassum, M., Lippman, U. S., Schwartz, R., and Slocum, B. A comparison of middle and lower class families in treatment at a child guidance clinic. *American Journal of Orthopsychiatry*, 1968, **38**, 814–822.

Strodbeck, F. L. Husband-wife interaction over revealed differences. *American Sociological Review*, 1951, **16**, 468–473.

Strodbeck, F. L. The family as a three person group. *American Sociological Review*. 1954, **19**, 23–29.

Strodbeck, F. L. Family interaction values and achievement. In D. C. McClelland et al. (Eds.), *Talent and society.* Princeton, N.J.: Van Nostrand, 1958.

Tanner, W. P., Jr., and Swets, J. A. A decision making theory of visual detection. *Psychological Review*, 1954, **61**, 401–409.

Thomas, A., Chess, S., and Birch, H. G. *Temperament and behavior disorders in children.* New York: New York University Press, 1968.

Tighe, L. S. and Tighe, T. J. Discrimination learning: two views in historical perspective. *Psychological Bulletin,* 1966, **66**, 353–370.

Tolman, E. C. Studies in spatial learning: II. Place learning versus response learning. *Journal of Experimental Psychology,* 1946, **36**, 221–229.

Towle, C., "The social worker," in Symposium: the treatment of behavior and personality problems in children. *American Journal of Orthopsychiatry,* Oct., 1930, **1**.

Truax, C. B. Effective ingredients in psychotherapy: An approach to unraveling the patient-therapist interaction. *Journal of Counseling Psychology,* 1963, **10**, 256–263.

Wallach, M. S. and Strupp, H. H. Dimensions of psychotherapists' activity. *Journal of Consulting Psychology,* 1964, **28**, 120–125.

Warren, J. R. Birth order and social behavior, *Psychological Bulletin, 1966,* **65**, 38–49.

Waters, E. and Crandall, V. J. Social class and observed maternal behavior from 1940 to 1960. *Child Development,* 1964, **35**, 1021–1032.

Watzlawick P., Beaver, J. H., and Jackson, D. D. *Pragmatics of human communication.* New York: Norton & Co., 1967.

Weakland, J. H. The "double-bind" hypothesis of schizophrenia and three party interaction. In D. D. Jackson (Ed.), *The etiology of schizophrenia.* New York: Basic Books, 1961.

Whorf, B. L. *Language, thought and reality.* Cambridge, Mass: MIT Press, 1956.

Winer, B. J. *Statistical principles in experimental design.* New York: McGraw-Hill, 1962.

Winter, W. D. and Ferreira, A. J. (Eds.). *Research in family interaction: Readings and commentary.* Palo Alto, Calif.: Science and Behavior Books, Inc., 1969.

Zax, M. and Cowen, E. L. Research on early detection and prevention of emotional dysfunction in young school children. In C. D. Spielberger (Ed.), *Current topics in clinical and community psychology,* Vol. I. New York: Academic Press, 1969.

Author Index

Strodtbeck, F. L., 13, 71
Strupp, H. H., 174
Suci, C. J., 18, 237
Summer, D., 181

Tannenbaum, P. H., 18, 237
Thomas, A., 182
Towle, C., 165
Truax, C. B., 153

Urban, H. B., 156

Vogel, J. L., 174

Wallach, M. S., 174

Walters, R. H., 105, 115
Warren, J. R., 28
Waters, E., 72
Watzlawick, P., 11
Waxler, N. E., 112
Weakland, J. H., 86, 109
White House Conference on Children,
    25
Whiting, J. W., 105
Wilson P., 26
Winer, B. J., 248, 275
Winter, W. D., 11, 13, 138
Wolfe, D. K., 71

Zax, M., 14

Subject Index

grade changes in, 174-175
lesser effectiveness of, 181-183
playground rating changes in, 180
similarity to parent counseling, 171, 200
Year I-Year II comparisons, 159-160,
173-174
Classroom behavior, observer ratings in, 126,
128-129, 158, 178-179, 225
Clinician experience levels, as related to
treatment outcomes, 173-174
as related to utilization of services, 159,
160, 161, 162-163
Clinicians, characteristics of, 161-162,
Table 23, 288
Cognitive emphasis in Information Feedback, 6, 175, 176, 177
Cognitive redefinition, 9
Commitment of authors as consultants,
relationship to treatment outcomes,
174
Communication, accuracy, 16, 88, 89, 92,
141
channels in, 224
inconsistency in, 5
interpersonal, 11. See also Family
communication task and Conflicting
messages
Community, orientation of Information
Feedback for work in, 231
parent involvement in, 60-61, 69, 73, 75
school relationships with, 148
Conduct grades, 23, 27-28, 33, 170, 171,
179
Conflict, child-adult, 62-63, 64, 120, 124,
133, 135, Table 24, 289
marital, 60-61, 66, 67, 132, 133
peer, 62, 64, 120
Conflicting messages, 109, 110, 111-112,
113, 115, 136, 140, 224. See also
Videotape study 2
Conforming behavior, 125, 144
Consent, parental, to clinic, 206
to schools, 155
Constructive behavior, 120, 125
Control children, 1, 20. See also Nonreferred
families, 20, 162, 166
Coping abilities, as focus in Information
Feedback, 4
Criteria, for matching control children, 1,
20
for referral, 154-155
for sample selection, 15
Crying, 54, 62, 63, 65, Table 24, 289

Data, naturalistic, 15, 223, 226
Decision making, parental patterns, 55, 60-
61, 66, 69, 73, 74, 75, 76
Defensive reactions, 5, 209

Demographic data, 1, 20
Dependency, child, 5, 31, 72, 75-76,
Table 24, 289
Dependent relationships in treatment, 176,
231
minimized in Information Feedback, 153,
155, 202, 203
Developmental levels, 67, 120
Dimensions, see Interpersonal behavior,
dimensions of
Directing behavior, in children, 63, 98, 103,
124-125
in fathers, 62, 63, 65, 98-100, 102, 104,
106, 108, 115, 136, 219
as an interpersonal dimension, 18, 38, 55,
68, 95-96
in mothers, 64, 65, 97, 131, 133, 134,
135, 136, 138
Directive interventions, 7, 175
Disciplinary techniques, fathers', 61-63,
70-71
mothers', 63-64, 71-72
Disruptive behavior, 30, 121, 126, 127
Distractibility, see Poor attention control
Disturbed children, see Referred children
Divergent behavior, 126, 127
Double-bind hypothesis, 109, 111, 136
Drop-outs, case illustrations, 184, 190-191,
194-195
within each treatment group, 163-164,
165
Dyads, parent-child, 94, 247

Ecological factors, 20
as related to psychological problems, 11
Educational level, of parents, Table 7, 272
Effectiveness, interpersonal, 52, 67-68, 120,
121, 124, 178, 230, Table 24, 289
Emotional-expressive behavior, 132, 138-
139, 147
Environmental emphasis in this study, 6,
11, 146, 227
Environments, differences for actor and
observer, 8
differences in home and school, 1, 11,
14, 148, 226
interpersonal, 1, 2
role in child behavior, 4-7, 11, 141, 146-
147, 148, 153, 226, 227, 270
Ethical considerations, 14, 92-93
Ethnic characteristics of sample, 1, 20
overlap with SEL, 21, 222
Evaluation, as an interpersonal dimension,
18, 38, 44, 55, 68, 95-108
for children, 98-99, 104, 107, 120,
124-125, 131
for fathers, 62, 65, 68, 98-100, 101,
104, 107, 108, 115, 136

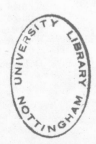